C0-AWE-479

Medicine & Society In America

Medicine & Society In America

Advisory Editor

Charles E. Rosenberg
Professor of History
University of Pennsylvania

THE
Married Lady's Companion,
OR
POOR MAN'S FRIEND.

BY SAMUEL K. JENNINGS

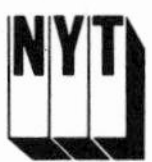

ARNO PRESS & THE NEW YORK TIMES
New York 1972

Reprint Edition 1972 by Arno Press Inc.

LC# 77-180580
ISBN 0-405-03957-3

Medicine and Society in America
ISBN for complete set: 0-405-03930-1
See last pages of this volume for titles.

Manufactured in the United States of America

THE

Married Lady's Companion,

OR

POOR MAN'S FRIEND.

IN FOUR PARTS.

I. An address to the Married Lady, who is the Mother of Daughters.
II. An address to the newly Married Lady.
III. Some important hints to the Midwife.
IV. An essay on the management and common diseases of children. To which will be added a short note on fever

BY SAMUEL K. JENNINGS.

Second edition, revised, corrected and enlarged by the Author.

The fear of the Lord prolongeth days ; but the years of the wicked shall be shortened.—PROV. X. 27.

PUBLISHED BY LORENZO DOW.

J. C. Totten, printer, No. 155 Chatham-street, New-York.

1808.

ADVERTISEMENT.

AS the medical part of this compilation was principally intended for the poor, and such other families as cannot conveniently obtain the aid of physicians, the author did not think it necessary to name the work from which each thought is extracted—He cheerfully and thankfully acknowledges himself indebted to the writings of Doctors Cullen, Rush, Darwin and others ; and in a very special manner to Dr. Denman's treatise on the diseases of women. It was his chief ambition, to feel himself conscious of benevolent intentions, whatever might be the reception of his work.

Since the publication of the first edition of this work, a copy has been submitted to the inspection of Dr. Rush. The Doctor thought proper to speak favorably of the performance, and to recommend it to such families as live in country places, or in places where skilful physicians are not easily obtained.

As the author has no pecuniary interest whatever in the edition which is now offered to the public, he feels himself at liberty to make an apology to the purchasers of the first.

In the first place, he was in greater haste in ushering it into the world than he would have been, had fame or interest been his principal object. But he was too often obliged to be an eye-witness to the dreadful ravages committed on the health and lives of women and children, by a number of self-conceited wretches, who seemed to be ignorant of the mischief they were doing in the world. These he wished to correct without delay.

In the second and last place he would observe, that his professional engagements were so considerable, that it was impossible for him to avoid delay, and yet be minutely correct—He was therefore contented with setting forth, in an intelligible manner, the great truths he intended, without much regard to elegance of style.

The present edition is intended to be a good deal more correct than the former, and is enriched with considerable additions.

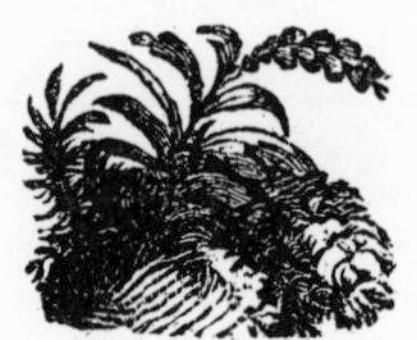

Part First.

Addressed to the married Lady who is the mother of daughters.

CHAPTER I.

INTRODUCTION.

MADAM,

AS a person much in the habit of thinking, you have often pitied the *silly creatures*, who rush into the bands of wedlock without duly considering the consequences. You are deeply sensible, that, on the mother's conduct and example is depending not only her own happiness, but also the well being of her children, and of her children's children, down to the latest generation.

I am secure of your attention then, while I state a few things, intended to assist you, in the important business of rightly instructing your daughters in the way to health and happiness.

If every woman were properly qualified, and would faithfully perform her duty in bringing up her children; their virtuous affections might be so confirmed, their disposition to vice so effectually subdued, that, the greatest revolution in the morals and health of the world, would be the consequence.

"Train up a child in the way he should go, and when he is old, he will not depart from it," says Solomon.

A sound mind in a sound body, will never fail to make her who is blest with them, as happy as is allowed of God to man in this world.

That these may be the lot of your daughters, is much more in your power than many are willing to believe. To bring them about however, it requires much pains and never ceasing diligence.

The weight of the task is thought by some, a sufficient excuse for neglecting it. But I hope the sincerity of your regard for your daughters' happiness has long since led you to undertake it as far as you were able, and prepared your mind, gladly to receive any assistance which may be offered you for its accomplishment.

CHAPTER II.

FUNDAMENTAL PROPOSITIONS.

1. HEALTH, MORALITY, and RELIGION, are mutually and essentially dependent on each other. For as sound health cannot be continued without good morals, so neither can sound morals be preserved without religious sentiment.

2. Our children are committed to our care in a state of infancy, that, we may so regulate their food, cloathing, exercise, and manner of thinking, as most effectually to prepare them for *health* and *happiness*.

3. While yet in their infant state, we perceive, they have all the passions to urge them into action, but they require much time and pains to gain that experience, which is necessary for the regulation of passion, which is too seldom gained even with riper years.

4. Hence I draw the two following conclusions, First, God wisely designed, that the reason and experience of parents, should be employed in the government of their children through the whole course of their infancy.

5. 2d, If parents do not use every possible exertion, and through neglect, their children should take a wrong direction, as parents

they are accountable for the injury done to their offspring, and as trustees, they are bound to answer to that society of which they are members, for all the consequent mischief brought upon the public.

6. The little bodies of our children first demand our care, in as much as a certain growth must take place before the mind unfolds itself.

7. We proceed however, but a short distance with our charge, before the task becomes a complicated one. Their minds quickly claim attention.

8. It is therefore important, that we should set out on such a plan, as may readily adapt itself to both these considerations, viz. The establishment of a sound *constitution of the body*, and the formation of the *virtuous affections of the mind.*

CHAPTER III.

IMPORTANCE OF EXERCISE FOR ESTABLISHING A GOOD CONSTITUTION.

The propensity of children to be in constant action, as well as the experience of mankind in all ages, sufficiently proves the importance of exercise of body, for establishing and preserving a good constitution.

The same experience has proved, that this exercise must be regularly continued, in order to make it effectual to such an important end.

I must therefore urge upon you the necessity of using all proper means, for forming in your daughter habits of industry. Look around among your female acquaintance, and see where is the greatest share of good health. Is it the lot of the rich and luxurious, who spend much of their time in bed, who take no exercise, but that of an occasional flight in the chariot or coach ? Let their pale countenance, their feeble arm, and bloated flesh answer for them !

No madam, the God of nature has fixed his firm decree, that indolence and health shall not dwell together. Shall I direct you in your search after health ?

Go see the blooming maid, dextrously whirling the useful wheel, cleaning and adjusting the furniture, regulating the wardrobe, directing in the kitchen, superintending the dairy. How cheerfully does she spend the day ! How sweet is her food ! How soft and pleasant her bed, when at an early hour she reclines herself to rest !

Not tired of inaction, her time hangs not heavy on her hand. She seeks no party to hide her from herself. Conscious of having spent the day in useful employment, she feels a sweet composure which the idler never knew.

Let these reflections suffice to prove, that industry best secures the greatest share of health.

But how are you to establish this industrious disposition? It is not enough for you occasionally to say in your daughters' hearing "*Industry is a fine thing*," "*Every body ought to work*," "*Indolence is shameful and is justly followed by beggary.*" These are all true, but nothing is more common with the most indolent, than frequent declamation of this sort.

You must set the example madam, you must diligently employ yourself in some valuable business, and then encourage your daughter to imitate you.

How often you have been pleased to extacy, when the little creature, even at three years old, would set down, patiently endeavouring to handle your scissors, your needles, or your thimble! How you have been amused, to see her little fingers trying faithfully to work up a bit of pastry!

Might not these hints be considered strong intimations of what is your duty? The case is plain. If you will take proper advantage of *this imitative disposition*, you may readily form in your child *what habit* you please.

Have you never seen an instance, where this favorable time for instruction was lost through neglect, through slothfulness, or through love of pleasure? Can you, madam, lay your hand upon your own heart, and in candor and truth say you have not been remiss? What followed? The little pratler for want of proper employment, turned her attention wholly from the business of the house, to sport at large in the field, and to indulge in dissipating plays. She lost her fondness for every thing useful, and would regret the loss of a few minutes from her play, even if called upon to prepare her own dress!

I do not mean that misses should be constantly kept in the house, nor too closely confined to the same thing. Nothing could be more pernicious to their health. Such conduct would subject them to vapours, hysterics, and all the train of hypochondriacal affections.

The design of the argument is, to urge upon you the propriety of introducing early into your family, habits of regularity. So soon as your daughter can perform any kind of business, fix for her regular times, and let her perform her task duly and daily. *And as often as you can do it with any shadow of truth, you will find it beneficial to give her a certain degree of praise. It is highly improper to degrade her, either publicly or privately.*

When exercise out of doors is thought necessary, let her be engaged in something which will keep up her attention, and yet let it be entirely agreeable.

I know it is advised by some, that girls should be indulged to sport and romp about at pleasure. It is not my design at present pointedly to deny it. But after they arrive at a certain age, I must insist on a proper regulation of those sports, both as to time and duration. And this of course will be the mother's task. Now what lady of discretion will neglect useful employment, to regulate the plays of children? Would it not be much more convenient, and consistent with her interest, to superintend some profitable engagement?

Suppose, for instance, your daughter were occasionally led to the garden, where she should have her proper lot of ground assigned her, for the cultivation of plants and flowers; and were thus taught so much of botany, as has reference to kitchen and ornamental purposes while she was exercising her body.

Might not this be a tolerable substitute for

romping and tearing about? Might not judicious mothers, who would make it their study, devise many plans like this, for forming habits of business and industry, to the exclusion of indolence and dissipation?

The greatest attention is necessary if you would succeed in this important business.—Do not object and say, the engagements of your family will not afford time or leisure for these things. Pray, tell me if you are able, *what mighty work you have to do*, which is of more importance than that of rightly bringing up your children.

Suppose you are able, by your neglect of this duty, to lay up a few more pounds.—When she comes to be a woman, a mistress of a family, and a mother of children, will that pittance of saving be of as much consequence to her, as a knowledge of business, and a willingness and ability to perform such business would have been?

But I am not disposed to grant that any such addition will be gained. Suppose for instance, you were willing to adopt the plan proposed, regularly dividing the time, so as to devote a certain number of hours daily, to reading and improving your daughter's mind; a certain number of hours to sewing, knitting or spinning; a certain number of hours to the business of the kitchen, dairy, &c.

keeping her constantly with you, and instructing her as you proceed in every branch of your engagements. Would you not execute more useful business in the course of the year, than you now do in the common bustling way? And even granting, that, some less was executed at the first, would not the aid of your daughter, who would on this plan quickly be prepared to assist you, more than make good the loss? Certainly it would: But it must also be granted, that your daughter's happiness will be infinitely more enhanced, by the effects which regularity will have on the state of her mind, than by any pecuniary consideration. However important therefore, you may think your business, every instance of neglect in her education is a proof, either of your want of information inducing an error in judgment, your want of industry, or your want of maternal affection.

It is true there are some in the world, who think much of themselves, and who may be highly esteemed by others like themselves, whose chief study it is, how to be *genteelly idle*, and who of course consider it a disgrace to be thus regularly employed. I expect however you will join me in pitying their weakness, for you cannot withhold your admiration, when you see a sweet little miss, regularly employed, handsomely preparing a room, dressing a table, and as your phrase is *putting things to rights*, taking pleasure chiefly in her business ! For my own part I confess, she seems to me as far superior to the ignorant, indolent, whining fool, as real worth and usefulness, is to insignificance and emptiness.

Inasmuch then, as regular exercise is important to the establishment and preservation of good health, as it is conducive to wealth and respectability, you surely are determined to adopt some plan to keep your daughter constantly employed. If you are not, and the sweet child should be cursed with a sickly constitution, merely from the want of sufficient firmness and attention on your part, how will you answer for it ? As a friend to mankind, I charge you to consider well the consequences. Do your duty as a mother, and you shall receive your just reward.

CHAPTER IV.

IMPORTANCE OF THE VIRTUOUS AFFECTIONS.

How great soever the pains necessary for confirming habits of industry, equal care must be taken for the cultivation of the virtuous affections. For without them, nothing can secure happiness to your daughter.

Mildness, Cheerfulness, Benevolence, Affection, &c. are so essential to the character of an amiable woman, that she who is destitute of these must be intolerable.

However severe you may think the sentence, you are responsible for the disposition of your child ; because by patient attention, and proper example, you may form it aright.

" *You are acquainted with an elderly lady, who is very peevish, ill-natured, restless, envious and unhappy. She has daughters too ; and they are as much like their mother as they can be.*" The thing is common, there is as much a family temper as there is a family likeness. An ill tempered woman, in almost every instance, shall have ill tempered children, and so the plague is handed down from generation to generation.

I perceive you will ask leave to excuse the poor woman, who is unhappy in an ill natured husband. This is indeed a serious difficulty. But the iniquity of the man, can by no means make atonement for the fault of his wife. She may do a great deal by a strict observance of her duty. The business of the man, frequently calls him abroad. The mother has the best opportunity to mould the tempers of her children. The same position of course still recurs upon you, " that every mother is in a very great degree responsible for the disposition of her children." To give you as special aid on this head as possible, I will offer a short essay on some of the most important passions.

CHAPTER V.

OF LOVE.

Love indulged without success, sometimes produces hypochondriacal affections, hysterics, fevers and death. Custom forbids the female to make suit to the male. Whether such a custom may not be founded in error, is not my business at present to enquire. It is now so firmly established, that the ladies are under the necessity of accommodating themselves to it.

They should therefore be able at all times to govern themselves with prudence. And every thing which may have a tendency to inflame this passion, ought to be cautiously avoided. Two things I will mention as being particularly pernicious.

And first, Idleness. " Every person who recollects his past conduct, may be satisfied, that, the hours of idleness have always proved the hours most dangerous to virtue.— They provoke the rise of criminal passions, lead to the suggestion of guilty pursuits, and to the formation of designs which in their issue bring disquiet and bitterness to the remainder of life.

"Sloth is like a slowly flowing, putrid stream which stagnates in the marsh, breeds venomous animals, and poisonous plants, and infects with pestilential vapours the whole country round it. Having once tainted the soul, it leaves no part of it sound."*

Idleness constantly nourishes the passions, and it must be very difficult, if not impossible, for her who is pampered in idle luxury to regulate that powerful propensity of which this chapter treats. The importance of industry for the preservation of health, has already been urged. I must however again speak of it as of the greatest moment for the government of passion. By forming those habits of order at which I have hinted, every thing may be met in its own place, and your daughter may constantly find innocent and useful employment for time. She will never be at a loss how to dispose of her hours, or to fill up life agreeably.

Such a plan only, can answer well the situation of an unmarried lady. On any other, she must be constantly perplexed, with all

---

* Dr. Blair.

the imaginations, which attend idleness and dissipation.

Secondly, Reading novels and romances. The unwarrantable amours and intrigues, which fill up most works of this kind, cannot fail to raise propensities the most unfriendly to virtuous continence. "Evil communication corrupts good manners." And to indulge the imagination in contemplating such amours, cannot differ but in degree, from associating with the hero or heroine of the play. Besides, the examples of human excellence, as displayed in most of their fine characters, do no where exist in real life.—Of course the unfortunate girl, who has formed an opinion of her lover from one of those highly coloured pictures, is at length disappointed, disgusted and miserable.

Better sentiments may be collected from other books, and you will be wise to commit your novels to the flames, rather than to the hands of your daughter.

Furthermore, when you seriously consider, that it is possible your daughter should run away with some worthless fellow, if her inclination should not accord with your judgment and advice, you will see that every precaution ought to be taken to regulate her mind on this important subject.

Begin in time to inculcate sentiments proper for her safety. Teach her that, it is im possible for a young impassioned miss to judge of man's merit. That it is far more properly the province of the parent.

Make it a rule of your house, *That no man shall pay his addresses to your daughter, without first explicitly obtaining permission from her father and yourself.* Impress on her mind the necessity and propriety of such a rule, that she may learn to consider any man an enemy, who would presume to speak on the subject of love without having regularly submitted to it.

Be careful also to secure your daughter's confidence. It is frequently the case, that, young ladies by confiding in their acquaintance, receive bad advice, are led to adopt dangerous measures, and are involved in ruin. Sometimes too, not having a confidant acquaintance, and not being disposed to confide in their mothers, they languish in secret, to the destruction of their health and happiness. These evils might be prevented, if mothers would take the proper steps to gain such confidence with their daughters, as to know all their distresses, and hear all their secrets.

It is furthermore possible, notwithstanding every precaution, that, a young lady should fix her affection upon some gentleman who has never thought proper to place himself within her power. Should this happen to your daughter, what could be done, if she dare not intrust you with a knowledge of her case? Whereas if you knew her inclination, you might adopt measures either to prevent or accomplish her wishes, as might be tho't most prudent. An instance of this sort may happen without disgrace.

"In one of the lower counties of Virginia, a young gentleman of agreeable address, excellent morals, and charming disposition, happened to reside in the family of a wealthy and respectable man, who was blessed with an amiable daughter. Although his great worth had secured to him the esteem of the whole family, whilst the young lady seemed to repose the utmost confidence in his friendship; yet as his fortune was very moderate, he dare not indulge a thought of gaining her affection. Several gentlemen of the first distinction waited on her with offers of marriage, but she very politely dismissed them all, 'till at length her parents were anxiously apprehensive, that, she must have formed a resolution never to marry. This worthy young man was particularly solicitous on her account, for he had considered some of the offers to be very advantageous. At the request of her friends, he therefore cheerfully undertook to enquire into the cause of her conduct, so apparently strange. With difficulty he extorted from her a confession, that her love was fixed upon another. It was then determined that he should continue the negociation, and if possible obtain a knowledge of the person. For some days she persisted to withhold the desired information. But at length yielding to his solicitude, she directed him to the 7th verse of the XII ch. of the second book of Samuel for a determinate answer. With haste he ran to his bible, and opening the place, to his astonishment and joy, he read, "and Nathan said unto David *thou art the man.*" They were happily married a short time after the discovery, and perhaps to this day are living in harmony."

Should a similar case occur, in which the young gentleman is not so easily gained, the friends of the young lady might use the influence of some worthy acquaintance to bring about a match, and there could be no impropriety in the measure.*

But if the object cannot be obtained, and

* From having still more maturely considered the delicacy of such a case, I am the more persuaded of the propriety of this instruction. It too often happens, that ladies failing of their own proper choice, are at length married from considerations of prudence, and what not, and are ever afterwards unhappy.

the passion is of the more violent kind, a fever will be the consequence. For the removal of this fever, blood letting and blistering are advised. These remedies frequently remove the passion together with the fever.

If the case be of the more moderate sort, the patient will probably talk incessantly of the beloved object, or will be too cautiously silent. Will sigh often. Will be unable to sleep. And will frequently retire into solitude, especially by moon light.

For the cure here, let the company of the object of affection be carefully avoided. A long journey through some pleasant country, would most effectually answer this purpose. All hope of success must be removed, and a decent resentment should be raised in its stead. In the mean time, her condition should be carefully concealed from all persons not immediately interested.

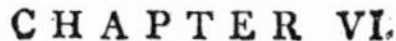

CHAPTER VI.

GRIEF.

Excessive grief is seldom the lot of misses. But the associations which most effectually prevent it in maturer years, are to be formed in infancy and youth. If you use every exertion to raise your daughter's expectations of the pleasures of the world, the first considerable disappointment will be sufficient to destroy her health, peace, and perhaps her life.

But if you begin early to teach her, that earthly things are fleeting. That " God has stamped the mark of uncertainty on all the comforts of this life, to teach man that his true happiness dwells not here, but is risen." By such lessons properly inculcated, her mind will be prepared to meet the loss of a friend, or any other misfortune, with composure.

Perhaps you may say this is preaching.—Call it by what name you please, it is truth, and therefore deserves your regard. It implies the necessity of Religion, and of the prospects which religion brings to view, for support under the calamities of life. Your daughter is now a blooming maid, but if your wishes are accomplished, she will shortly be a wife, and the mother of children.—She must of course, be liable to become a widow, and to be bereft of those children.—Even granting it as a certain thing, that she shall live and be blest to see them grow up and multiply around her, yet she must suffer considerable apprehension in every instance of her pregnancy. And if she have the affection for her children, necessary to make her happy in them, as often as any one of them complains, she anticipates the pangs she would feel on its death. Add to these, the certainty of being at last separated from the whole at a stroke. How gloomy the prospect! How destructive to her bliss!—Let her be taught, that in this world we have but the beginning of our existence. That friends must part for a season here, but part to meet again, where all sorrow shall be done away. Then she will rationally enjoy the comforts of life. "*Using the world as not abusing it*, *remembering* daily *that the fashions thereof pass away*." This view of things, and this only, can sustain her in the time of distress, and is therefore of the greatest importance to her health.

For grief indulged, spoils digestion and destroys the appetite, hence from want of proper nourishment, the whole system is relaxed, the spirits sink, the circulation becomes irregular, inducing a train of formidable diseases; as fainting, swooning, falling-sickness, apoplexy, palsy and the whole train of hypochondriacal affections, madness, and death.

Should any misfortune happen to your daughter, as the loss of a friend, or a disappointment in love, begin speedily to bring consolation to her mind. Place her among cheerful, but sober companions. Levity instead of lessening, will but increase her distress. The conversation should turn upon important, yet interesting subjects. Her employment should be calculated to keep up attention. If it be convenient have her instructed in some art, which will employ her skill to the utmost. Sleep may be procured by the help of the tincture of opium. Her appetite and strength may be restored by exercise, and the medicines proper for strengthening the stomach ; as bark, wine, steel, &c.

CHAPTER VII.

ANGER.

Anger of all the passions, least becomes female delicacy. And one would expect, the love of beauty, so common to the sex, would induce them to guard against an emotion, so unfriendly to the symmetry of the human countenance. That fulness and redness of the face and eyes, that foaming of the mouth, and unequaled volubility of the tongue, that clenching of the fists and stamping of the feet, attendant on excessive anger, may correspond with the character of a drunken bully, a waggoner, or sailor, but never with the angelic sweetness, which we expect to meet in the amiable woman. "Be angry and sin not. Let not the sun go down upon thy wrath," is an express command of God by Paul.

Be careful often to represent to your daughter, the sinfulness of excessive anger. Shew her how impolite it is! How degrading to the dignity of a lady! How destructive to her beauty! How pernicious to her respectability and happiness. Prevail with her, at all times to reflect when her anger is about to rise and be silent. For every indulgence in loud scolding and railing against the offender, will serve to increase her rage. To effect these things, it will be necessary for you to gain her highest respect in time of her infancy, by setting before her proper examples. Parents, and especially you who are a mother, cannot possibly be too particular on this point.

You ought never to let your daughter know, that you can be excited by any means to indulge this hateful passion. Shew her, that no offence can transport you beyond the bounds of a descreet woman. That you consider it more noble to forgive, than to resent an offence.

Inform her, that in many instances anger

has brought on the most dangerous diseases, as hysterics, convulsion, paleness, tremors, sickness, puking of bile, fainting, syncope, apoplexy and death.

And surely, when she is taught, that her beauty, her respectability, her happiness and her very life may be destroyed by this indelicate passion, she will strive to prevent its indulgence from becoming habitual.

To succeed the more effectually, if she should be of an irrascible constitution, she should be put upon a milk and vegetable diet only.*

CHAPTER VIII.

FEAR.

Fear perhaps, has injured the health of the ladies more frequently than any of the passions. It is indeed ridiculous to hear the screams of a modern fine lady, at the appearance of a catterpillar, spider, any insect or

* The benefit to be derived from abstinence was considered by the Great Author of the Christian religion and his disciples. Temperance in all things is stated as being essential in forming true happiness.— And fasting and prayer were found effectual in keeping the *body*, that is the passions, in proper subjection.

other harmless and insignificant object. Yet I believe, if once the habit of being easily affrighted is completely formed, any such trivial object, may prove sufficient to bring on hysterics, convulsions, madness and death.

How injudiciously! How unfriendly do mothers act towards their daughters, when they retail to them stories of ghosts, hobgoblins, and faries? of the mighty feats wrought of witches in the form of cats? Their strange power to injure their fellow creature, &c.!! And how dangerous to join in tricks to give them alarm!!

Instead of these things, the greatest care should be taken, to moderate and subdue a timorous disposition. I am induced to believe, that if children were never told there is danger in the dark, they would have no more fear in the night than in the day. In proof of this opinion, I state it as a fact, that the children of hunters and others towards the west, will turn out into the wild forest at any time of the night, fearing nothing.

The great importance of these precautions will furthermore appear, when you reflect on the peculiar condition of a delicate lady with a cowardly imagination, in a state of pregnancy. The terrible apprehensions which haunt her day and night have brought about more deaths, than parturition itself. By such continual terror, they seldom escape abortion, and if they do escape such debility is induced, as exposes them to actual danger in childbed, *and sometimes to a consumption which always has debility for its predisposing cause.*

But the peculiar diseases of ladies of this description, are not confined to the times of pregnancy. The very possibility of sickness and death, is a continual source of the most destructive terror, so that through fear of death, they are all their life-time subject to bondage.

Wisdom requires, that we should adapt our conduct and our feelings to our condition. In this consists our chief happiness, and our capacity for this, is the foundation of our accountability. To prepare your daughter for this great work, daily impress on her mind, the importance of a firm reliance on the protection of Providence. Use your utmost ability, both by precept and example, to engage her in the cultivation of such devout sentiments and religious practices as are necessary, for acquiring and preserving confidence in God's mercy and favor. By these means and by these only, she will be able to overcome the fear of death, and gain that state of composure so important to the ladies. I once heard a physician of some note declare, (himself being very irreligious at the same time) 'that religion was an essential part of a lady's education.' Their particular ills, make particular aid necessary for their support.

CHAPTER IX

JOY.

Joy is an emotion, which seldom produces any ill effects. In some instances however, when great and sudden, it produces fainting and swooning. In a case of this kind, let the patient be erected in a sitting posture, then sprinkle cold water, or vinegar and water in her face, and apply strong vinegar to her nose, and she will in most instances be speedily recovered. Such an accident might generally be prevented, if the absent friend, or joyful message, be prudently and gradually introduced.*

* Friction with the hand or flesh brush applied to the naked stomach, would sometimes be found useful, especially if ordinary means fail

CHAPTER X

ENVY.

Envy is a certain painful sensation, felt at seeing another's happiness. This is a base passion, and never fails to make wretchedly miserable, every lady over whom it has gained ascendency.

" Thou shalt love thy neighbor as thyself." The benevolence taught by this excellent precept of the gospel, is the proper preventative and cure for this hateful emotion.

If you will cultivate in yourself a disposition to *feel*, and of course to *express* congratulation, as often as you see your neighbor happy ; your daughter will readily drink in the same spirit. But if you indulge an envious disposition, she will learn with you, to be miserable as often as any one of her acquaintance is happy.

It is your privilege " to rejoice with those who rejoice." Possessing a benevolent disposition, you may enjoy the emotion attendant on any happy event, although it should not turn up in your favor exclusively. You may in this sense, partake of all your neighbor's success. If this temper of mind were made universal, what a vast addition would it bring to the present stock of human bliss !

CHAPTER XI

MALICE.

Malice is defined, 'a sincere wish for the injury of a fellow creature.' 'A thirst for vengeance.'

This emotion is a horrid departure from humanity. If you will cultivate a disposition to forgive any offence that may be offered you ; if you will use words and actions expressive of pity and compassion, towards every one who may injure your person, reputation, or property ; such a continued display of this virtuous affection, will insensibly lead your daughter into a similar forgiving temper. All malice, that passion so characteristic of the devil himself, would of course be excluded.

CHAPTER XII.

With these hints on the several passions, as a faithful mother strictly attentive to your daughter's happiness, you may pursue the subject at your leisure, and collect such further information as occasion may require, and as opportunity may serve.

By diligent observation, you may readily discover whether any of the passions have become too strong. Which ever it may be, use every exertion until it be properly subdued. By patient attention and perseverance, you will at length enjoy a daughter, who will be at once the delight of her acquaintance, the desire of men of worth, and an honor to her family. Blessed with happiness in herself, she will assist you in diffusing that inestimable treasure all around you, to your great consolation and unspeakable joy. If however, in consequence of neglect on your part, or of an incorrigible disposition on the part of your daughter, her passions are already become boisterous, bringing upon her criminality in the sight of God and man, advise her to betake herself to repentance and prayer. And if, through the rich mercy and grace of God, her sins be forgiven, and she be enabled under the influence of the spirit of truth, to bring her unruly passions into subjection, she will have abundant cause to rejoice in the God of salvation. I must conclude these observations on the passions, with a recommendation of the Holy Scriptures, as the best guide and source of information, in bringing about that happy disposition of soul, which will secure peace within your own breast, and respectability among your friends. In one word, without an experimental knowledge of the truth, as con tained in that book, I have no expectation, that you will set before your daughter the examples necessary to give you the weight and influence with your family, which are necessary for its successful instruction and happy government. If your daughter hrough your neglect or want of moral excellence, should be eursed with vicious disposition and habits, remember you will answer for it at the bar of God in the *great day*.

CHAPTER XIII.

TEMPERANCE IN EATING, &c.

A certain delicacy of person, is thought desirable by most women of fashion. They cannot bear the complexion of *health* because marked with *grossness*. To secure this delicate appearance, they are in the habit of starving their daughters, or compelling them to use such food as does not afford sufficient nourishment.

This is cruel and ridiculous conduct. It is *cruel* to deprive your child of the greatest earthly blessing, by conforming to a *ridiculous* opinion. As if a pale sickly countenance, is more beautiful than the bloom of health. The grand object I suppose is to marry her respectably. Now what man of common sense, would not more cheerfully connect himself with a healthful constitution, than enlist a nurse for life? Which is the more rational choice? A lady who has ability to take charge of a family, and assist in the management of an estate, or a valetudinarian, for the preservation of whose life, it would be necessary to expend an estate in the payment of nurses and doctors fees? Let common sense direct your conduct in this matter. Give your daughter enough of wholesome food.

But while you avoid one extreme, do not fall into another. Too full meals are always injurious. A plain simple manner of living is most safe and salutary. It will seldom happen that any decent person will eat too much of one dish. The desserts introduced for the second or third course of a feast, generally do the mischief. If therefore, this kind of parade be important to support the dignity of your table, take the necessary pains to prevent your daughter from injuring her health by loading her stomach with such a dangerous composition. It is far best for health, and would soon become most agreable, to make each meal of one dish only.— This kind of simplicity is unfashionable I acknowledge, but I must confine myself to truth whatever be the fate of fashion.

Dr. Buchan in his essay on this subject introduces the following quotation. 'For my part,' says Addison, 'when I behold a fashionable table, set out in all its magnificence, I fancy I see gouts, and dropsies, fevers and lethargies, with other innumerable distempers, lying in ambuscade among the dishes."

CHAPTER XIV.

Having given you some directions, for securing to your daughter a sound mind in a sound body, so far as it can be effected by management, &c. I now proceed, to consider the diseases to which she may sometimes be subject from accident, from constitutional defect, and the like, notwithstanding all your care. But that the instruction may be clear and distinct as possible, I must consider each one in a separate chapter.

CHAPTER XV.

MENSES.

There is a certain periodical evacuation which takes place with all healthy females beginning when they arrive at twelve or fifteen years of age, and continuing on till they are forty-five or fifty. This I shall call the *menses*. Perhaps this cannot properly be called a disease, as it is universal to the sex and as there cannot be health without it. You should begin in due time, to instruct your daughter in the conduct and management of herself at this critical time of life. A few lessons seasonably given may prevent much mischief.

But little attention is necessary, to know when this discharge is about to commence. There are particular symptoms which go before it and foretel its approach ; as a sense of heat and weight, with a dull pain in the loins, a swelling and hardness of the breasts, headache, loss of appetite, uncommon weakness of the limbs, paleness of the countenance, and sometimes a slight degree of fever. Whenever these symptoms appear about the age at which the menstrual flux usually begins to flow, every thing that might obstruct it, must be carefully avoided, and such means should be used as tend to bring it forward.

She should sit over the steams of warm water, bathing her feet at the same time in a vessel filled with the same, and so deep as to reach up to her knees. And she should drink freely of warm diluting liquors, such as weak flax-seed tea, mallows or balm teas. The most proper time for these things, is the evening, so that she may cover herself up warmly in bed after the bathing, and afterwards continue the drinks until bed time.

Some precautions, however, are necessary before the symptoms which usher in this discharge present themselves. For if she be closely confined about this time, and be not engaged in some active employment, which may give proper exercise to her whole body, she will become weak, relaxed, and sickly; her countenance will be pale and sallow, her spirits will sink, her vigor decline, and she becomes a valetudinarian for the remainder of her life.

It is often the case that the daughters of the fashionable and wealthy, who according to custom have been much indulged, entirely give themselves up to indolence at this critical time, and bring upon themselves such irregularity as renders them miserable for life.

We seldom meet with complaints from cold as it is commonly called, among active industrious girls, while on the contrary, the indolent and slothful are seldom freed from them.

A sprightly disposition, and an habitual cheerfulness, ought to be cultivated with all possible attention, not only as conducive to prevent obstructions, but as the best defence against vapours and hysterics.

The cheerfulness however which I here recommend, is not mere mirth and laughter. It is a calm and uniform serenity, which prepares a rational being thankfully and heartily to enjoy the real comforts of life. It is a peculiar spring which gives to the mind as much activity when in retirement or in the midst of daily engagements, as when in a ball room.

Towards this time, every thing which has a tendency to impair digestion, and derange the regular motions of the system, ought to be avoided; such as, eating largely of *trash*, tight clothes, loss of sleep, and excessive exercise. To this last we may generally affix dancing. Change of clothes, without proper regard being had to their degree of warmth, is frequently productive of mischief. Occasional exposure of the skin to cool air, if continued for a short time only, seldom does injury. But a great change in the clothes from warm to cool, is frequently very pernicious. Changes of this kind ought to be brought about in a gradual manner. I have known serious effects from too long exposure of the feet to wet and cold. Country girls frequently wade through the water, walk barefoot in the dew of the morning, and sit without doors for hours together in the evening, &c. Either of these acts may do irreparable damage, whether about the time of the first flowing of the menses, or at any time of its return.

Indeed such exposure, as at another time might produce no ill effects, may at this juncture be followed by irretrievable damage to her health.

CHAPTER XVI.

RETENTION OF THE MENSES.

After all your care it will sometimes happen, that the menses will not begin to flow at that period of life when they usually make their appearance. Should this be the case, and in consequence of their retention her health and spirits begin to decline, by no means be persuaded to confine her to her room, nor expect to restore her by heat and medicine only. Instead of confinement, carry her abroad into agreeable company, turn her attention to some interesting employment, let her eat plentifully of wholesome food, and promote its digestion by taking regularly a sufficient portion of exercise; and in most instances nature will do her own work, without any other assistance than that recommended at chap. XV.

Having pursued this plan a sufficient length of time without success, you will be at liberty to have recourse to medicines, and with this intention you may observe the advice under the head of obstructed menses, chap. XIX. Sometimes the retention is the consequence of an imperforated *hymen*. When this is the case, it may be felt with the finger, and must be pierced with a proper instrument. For this purpose a surgeon should be employed.

CHAPTER XVII.

DIFFICULTY OF MENSTRUATION WITH PAIN, &c.

When the monthly complaint comes on too slowly, attended with pain, the menstruation may be said to be difficult. In this case the patient commonly is subject to a coldness of the extremities, particularly of the feet, and to great general weakness. The cause of this complaint is nearly the same as that of an entire obstruction, and will therefore yield to the same treatment. Which see in the following chapter. But when the painful symptoms come on, bathe her lower extremities in warm water of about blood heat, to be continued half an hour, just before going to bed. On lying down, give from twenty-five to fifty drops of the tincture of opium.—Repeat this plan every night till the pains abate. Afterwards in the intervals, between the times of the discharge, pursue one of the plans advised in the following chapter, regulating your choice according to the prevailing symptoms of her case.

CHAPTER XVIII.

OBSTRUCTED MENSES.

If by alternate exposure to heat and cold, or by any other accidental means, the menses cease to flow, they are said to be obstructed.

There are different appearances in this disease, according to the state of the general system. I shall mark three variations for the sake of distinction.

The first is generally brought on by some kind of exposure or accident. In this case, there will be a sensible fullness or increased motion of the blood, producing a swimming and dull heavy pain of the head, which are increased on stooping down, a redness, a fullness, with a sense of weight across the eyes, an aversion to motion, an unusual sense of weakness and heaviness of all the limbs, and sometimes a bleeding at the nose, &c.

Where these, or most of these symptoms occur,

1st. Let blood from the foot ten or twelve ounces, to be repeated as occasion may require.

2d. Bathe her feet half an hour on going to bed.

3d. Then give a portion of calomel and aloes three grains of each. Syrrup of some kind may be added so as to form it into a pill or two, or so much as to make it of the consistence of honey. Continue the bath and calomel and aloes, for three successive nights.

If the disorder came on suddenly, and especially if she was a healthy girl, before the attack, you may use the lancet the more freely.

There is no danger from the use of calomel. The only necessary precautions are, to avoid improper exposure to cold and wet, and abstain from large draughts of cold water. And these would be equally necessary if no calomel were used. At the next period proceed a second time through the same course, viz. bleed, bathe, and give calomel and aloes for three successive nights, and if there be not something more amiss than what you call a *common cold*, she will probably be relieved. It might not be amiss however to repeat it a third time if necessary.

CHAPTER XIX.

OBSTRUCTION OF MENSES CONTINUED.

The second variation of this complaint is not in general so suddenly induced as the former, and for the most part seizes upon the indolent. The symptoms are, great paleness or rather yellowness and bloating of the face, difficulty or shortness of breathing, loathing of food, indigestion, disposition to eat chalk or marle, great weakness, quick and weak pulse, swelling of the feet and ankles, and in some instances a bloating of the whole body. Sometimes these symptoms attend a retention of the menses. In either case observe the following plan.

1. A dose of calomel at night. Say six grains. Afterwards repeat smaller doses, as three or four grains, two or three times, letting a few days intervene between each dose.

2. Bitters of camomile and orange peel steeped in boiling water, may be used a few days, gradually increasing their strength.

3. Then take rust of iron prepared, one ounce; gum myrrh one ounce;* nutmegs No. 2. or cinnamon half an ounce. The whole to be finely powdered, carefully mixed, and kept in a close vessel. If rust of iron cannot be had, the salt of steel will answer, using half the quantity. Of this preparation, if made with the rust of iron, six or eight grains may be taken from four to six times a day. If prepared with the salt of steel, four to six grains will be the dose. The portion of either ought to be varied according to circumstances. It excites a little sickness of the stomach. But if a puking or too violent sickness be excited, the dose may be lessened. On the other hand, if no considerable effects are observed, it may be enlarged.†

4. Regular exercise. As friction with a flesh brush or flannel, riding in a carriage or on horse-back, &c.

5. Rhubarb five grains united with opium half a grain, given every night when great costiveness does not forbid their use.

6. Flesh diet with wine and water, when no fever exists.

---

* If the gum myrrh be offensive it may be omitted, regulating the dose accordingly.

† Advantage is sometimes gained from enlarging the dose of iron to five or six times the quantity here stated.

7. And when she begins to regain her strength and colour, at every appearance of the pains which usher in the menstrual evacuation use the aid advised in chapter XVII.

CHAPTER XX.

OBSTRUCTION OF MENSES CONTINUED.

A third distinction is a mixed state of the disease. It is the consequence of debility induced by a complaint of some kind which goes before it. The discharge gradually lessens in quantity; becomes irregular, and at length disappears. It is a common mistake in cases of this kind, that all the existing complaints are the effects of the deficiency or absence of the menses. But the reverse of this is true. The obstruction is merely a symptom. In all these mixed cases, there is difficulty in making the proper distinctions, and therefore if convenient, it will be best to employ some physician of approved judgment. If however she decline in a gradual manner; is subject to dejection of spirits; to a want of appetite; to flashings of heat over the skin; to a small cough; to occasional flushings of one or both ch eks; and to a smarting or burning sensation in the external parts of generation, &c. You might be safe in introducing the following plan of treatment.

1. Draw a blister on the region of the stomach or between the shoulders, and repeat it after some days.

2. In the mean time let her drink freely of warm camomile tea, made pretty strong, beginning early in the morning while yet in bed, and continuing it the greater part of the day.

3. Having continued the camomile a week or two, give bitters made of orange peel steeped in boiling water.

4. Friction with flesh brush or flannel, with other moderate exercise as soon as she is able; as riding on horseback, or in a carriage, &c.

5. As she strengthens, add to the bitters a portion of the peruvian bark.

6. And finally the preparation of iron with wine and water as recommended in chap. XIX.

It may be observed however, that if iron in any case produces the headache attended with a sense of heat, and pain in the breast or side, it must be omitted. In that case it will probably become indispensably necessary to use the calomel in this case also, as advised in the preceding chapter.

7. When her strength is recovered and the symptoms indicating the approach of the menses present themselves, proceed as advised at chap. XVII.

8. Where there is smarting in the external parts of generation, bathe frequently with warm milk and water, and anoint with fresh butter or sweet oil. If by these or any other means her health is restored, her menses will return as a thing of course.

CHAPTER XXI.

IMMODERATE MENSES.

When the menses continue too long or come on too often for the strength of the patient, they are said to be immoderate. This most frequently happens to women of a soft delicate habit; to such as use tea and coffee too freely, and who do not take sufficient exercise. It is sometimes brought on by excessive fatigue, and this may happen to temperate and industrious women. In either case, its approach may be known by a pain in the loins and hips. Observe this symptom carefully and on its first appearance let a little blood from the arm, and it will generally prevent the attack for that time. But for the entire removal of it, observe the following directions.

1. So soon as it is known that this complaint is formed, it will be proper to bleed a little from the arm. There are but few instancces in which this might not be proper, in greater or lesser quantities.

2. If excessive labour brought on the disease, rest comes in as an essential remedy.

3. Cool air is highly proper. This may be applied by placing the patient in such a situation, that a current from a door or window may blow upon her.

4. Cloths weted in cold vinegar and water may be applied all over the groins, &c. to be changed as they become warm.

5. Cold flour in a large quantity applied immediately to the parts has sometimes succeeded in dangerous cases.

6. Cool drinks, as the decoction of nettle roots or of the greater comfry, &c,

7. If all these fail, repeat the bleeding.

8. Where too strong a motion of the arteries can be ascertained as the cause, it may generally be entirely removed by gentle bleeding and purging occasionally repeated.

9. If much weakness, paleness, and a disposition to bloat attend, give half a grain of opium every six hours, and at intervals of three and four hours, give twelve or fifteen

grains of an equal mixture of allum and gum kino.

10. Nauseate the stomach with small doses, from one to five grains of ipecacuanha.

11. Apply blisters to the wrists and ankles alternately.

12. In all delicate cases, after the removal of the disease for the time being, have recourse to the cold bath, exercise, friction with a flesh brush or flannel, &c. till her health is confirmed.

CHAPTER XXII.

FLOUR ALBUS, OR WHITES.

When a discharge of whitish matter flows instead of the menses, it is called the flour albus, or whites. If it be of long standing, it sometimes assumes a greenish or yellow complexion, becomes acrid, sharp, and corroding, and is highly offensive to the smell. When it happens to young women, it is in most cases a local disease. I mean by this, that it is seldom brought on by any general effection of the system, but is chiefly confined to the parts which are its seat. Indeed it is sometimes the case, that the menses are discharged entirely in this way.

For the cure, give her iron as in chap. XIX. but in most cases the gum myrrh may be left out of the composition. A decoction of pine buds, or the roots of pine, or what is better, turpentine in its soft state mixed with an equal quantity of honey. Of this mixture a teaspoonful may be taken three times a day. Or for those who can procure it, balsam capævi, twenty drops, in a little new milk, three times a day. Frequently cleanse the parts with milk and water. Sometimes an injection, made of sixty grains of white vitriol dissolved in a pint of spring or rain water, and thrown into the passage by the help of a syringe, three or four times a day, is a most effectual remedy.

And lastly, if ulcers attend, give two or three grains of calomel every third night, and touch the ulcers with a little blue mercurial ointment, or with an ointment of white or red percipitate of mercury.

Here it might be well to observe, that a disease in some decree similar to flour albus, or more commonly of a mixed kind, between this and immoderate menses, is sometimes the effect of a polypus, or excrescence from the inner surface of the womb. If therefore the discharge should continue after using the proper remedies, a polypus ought to be suspected, and a physician or surgeon should be called in to your aid.

CHAPTER XXIII

HYSTERICS.

Missess are sometimes subject to hysteric affections, about the time of their first menstuation. This is an unfortunate circumstance whenever it occurs, inasmuch as such will be liable to similar complaints for many years afterwards. A complete cure of this disease is seldom obtained, but there is some ground to hope for a recovery if the proper remedies be employed on the first attack, or before it is too deeply rooted in the system. This truly distressing complaint, puts on a great variety of shapes. It is called a *proteus* of diseases, imitating almost every disorder, to which the human body is subject. But I shall confine myself to the description of those symptoms which are most remarkable. The principal and discriminating marks, are the three following.

1. A peculiar kind of suffocation. This generally begins with a perception of a globe or ball rolling round, seemingly among the bowels, and rising up to the stomach and

throat, and there inducing strangling. This generally excites great alarm, with the most excruciating fear of immediate death. Consequently it will be attended with great paleness, and a profuse discharge of limpid urine.

2. An unusual gurgling of the bowels, as if some little animal were there in actual motion, with wandering pains, constituting cholic of a peculi r kind.

3. Frequent efforts to vomit without any evacuation. This is sometimes mistaken for a symptom of an inflamatory affection of the stomach, and other intestines. In this case there is always a great weakness of the stomach; a considerable degree of indigestion, and anxiety; and sometimes a difficulty of breathing, with alternate flashings of heat and chilly sensations, over different parts of the body. To these particular distinctions may be added alternate laughing and weeping, without any known or adequate cause, faintings, convulsions, and palpitation or fluttering of the heart. Hysterical convulsions may be distinguished from those of epilipsy, or common convulsions, by the great fear of dying, which is peculiar to hysterics.

For the cure observe the following plan.

1. On the first attack, if it be the consequence of difficult or obstructed menstruation, let blood freely from the foot, and this

the more certainly, if she was strong and healthy before the attack.

2. If the sense of suffocation be violent, apply strong vinegar or spirits of hartshorn to her nose. Bathe her feet in warm water, apply pretty severe friction to the region of her stomach, with a flesh brush or flannel. And in some instances a glyster of very cold water, affords instant relief.

3. After the fit goes off, have recourse to the instructions given in chaps. XVI, XVII, XVIII, &c. For if the difficulty or obstruction of the menses be the cause of the complaint, let the cause be removed and the effect will follow.

4. But if she were delicate and feeble before the attack, use the vinegar, or spirits of hartshorn, and warm bath to the feet, &c. as above, according to circumstances ; but be cautious about letting blood.

5. For the radical cure in this last case, apply a blister to the stomach, use friction nearly all over the skin. Give strong camomile tea to drink. Wine, bark and steel, as at chap. XIX. Riding on horseback, cheerful company, and interesting engagements, each in their place may be proper.

6. And in many instances, I have found great benefit from the use of the following pills, viz. Take assafetida half an ounce

Russian castor quarter of an ounce, opium quarter of an ounce. Carefully beat and thoroughly mix them together, and of the whole, make two hundred pills of equal size as nearly as may be. Of these, two or three may be given at night, and one or two in the morning.

7. Where the patient is subject to a costive habit, I have found advantage from the following composition. Aloes one ounce, assafetida half an ounce, Russian castor quarter of an ounce. The whole to make two hundred pills and taken as before, increasing or lessening the number, according to the state of the bowels.

8. The vitriolic ether, given from thirty to fifty drops in a cup of some kind of drink, sometimes affords instant relief, when the suffocation is considerable and distressing.—This article must be given speedily, to prevent its loss by evaporation, and must not be opened too near to a candle, because of its great readiness to take fire.

CHAPTER XXIV

*CESSATION OF THE MENSES.**

All women are alarmed at the time of the final cessation of the menses, believing that some ill consequences may follow. The truth is, that scarce one of a great number of women, suffer more than temporary inconvenience on that account. It must be acknowledged however, that if there be a disposition to disease in the constitution, and especially in the womb, it will proceed more rapidly when the menses cease, by being deprived of that local discharge by which they were before relieved. Many remedies have been advised to prevent, and correct the mischief, expected or supposed to exist. But the present mode of practice is, to bleed occasionally and give gentle cooling purges, as manna, cream of tartar or common purging salts, &c. avoiding all kinds of medicines and diet which are heating.

This practice is both rational and successful. I have found it a good way, to lessen

* Although it may seem a little irregular, to treat of the cessation of the menses, a disease of advanced life, in that part of the work designed for misses only, yet as it is under the head of menses, it must be admitted on the whole as regular.

the quantity of blood to be taken, in a gradual manner, so as to imitate as nearly as possible, the most regular cessation in the natural way.

END OF THE FIRST PART.

Part Second.

Addressed to the Newly Married Lady.

CHAPTER I.

INTRODUCTION.

MADAM,

YOU have happily allied yourself to the man for whom you leave your father's house, for whom you cheerfully forsake all the world besides. With him, as your protector and bosom friend, you promise yourself many endearing pleasures. You perceive that "Innocence, candor, sincerity, modesty, generosity, heroism and piety, express themselves with grace ineffable in every attitude, in every feature of the man you love."* You are therefore highly concerned how you may secure an equal share, and a permanent continuance of his affection and esteem. On

* St. Pierre

this point turns your future happiness or misery. Mutual love and tenderness properly preserved, secures to you the greatest earthly blessing. In proportion to the want or loss of these, you are miserable for life.— Although this consideration very much concerns your husband as well as yourself, yet I must be permitted to assure you, that you are most deeply interested. His engagements as a man, will necessarily keep up his attention. He will have frequent occasion to mix with agreeable and interesting company. His acquaintance will be extended, his amusements multiplied. He of course will have an asylum, should home become tiresome or disagreeable. But your house is your only refuge, your husband your only companion. Should he abandon you, solitude, anxiety and tears, must be your unhappy lot. You cannot fly for amusement to the race ground, to the chase, to the card table, or to the tavern. You cannot look out for a gallant, to whom you may impart your slighted love. You must either languish in bitterness, or learn to compose your feelings, by stoical indifference.

CHAPTER II.

PROPER CONDUCT OF THE WIFE TOWARDS HER HUSBAND.

1. As it is your great wish and interest, to enjoy much of your husband's company and conversation, it will be important to acquaint yourself with his temper, his inclination, and his manner, that you may render your house, your person and your disposition quite agreeable to him. By observing with accuracy, and guarding your words and actions with prudence, you may quickly succeed according to your wishes.

2. Here perhaps you ask, why so much pains necessary on my part? I will answer your question candidly. Your choice in forming the connexion, was at best a passive one. Could you have acted the part of a courtier and made choice of a man whose disposition might have corresponded precisely with yours, there would have been less to do afterwards. But under present circumstances, it is your interest to adapt yourself to your husband, whatever may be his peculiarities. Again, nature has made man the stronger, the consent of mankind has given him superiority over his wife, his inclination is, to claim his natural and acquired

rights. He of course expects from you a degree of condescension, and he feels himself the more confident of the propriety of his claim, when he is informed, that St. Paul adds his authority to its support. "Wives submit yourselves unto your own husbands, as unto the Lord, for the husband is the head of his wife."

3. In obedience then to this precept of the gospel, to the laws of custom and of nature, you ought to cultivate a cheerful and happy submission. "The way of virtue is the way of happiness." The truth of this maxim will be verified to you in your conformity to this duty. By such submission, you will secure to yourself the advantages of a willing obedience on the part of your husband to the counter part of Paul's command, "Husbands love your wives as your own flesh," & .*

4. The great attention and submission, practised by most men in time of courtship, are well calculated to raise in the female

* There are some women, who pluming themselves upon their great spirit, spurn at this instruction, and claim the right of "*superior equality*" with their husbands. In most instances they pay very dearly for their arrogance. If they secure a degrading obedience, they necessarily loose that tender and engaging fondness and attention, which every condescending wife is sure to receive from the man of good sense, taste and refinement.

mind, false expectation of an uniform continuance of the same officiousness after marriage. For the honey moon you may not be disappointed. But the charge of a family will soon teach any man, that he has something more to do than live a life of courtship. The discharge of his duty as a father, a friend, and a citizen, will gradually divert him in some degree from that punctilious attention to your person, with which you are so highly pleased.

5. Should you begin to discover this change, be careful to conduct yourself with discretion. By no means upbraid him, nor suffer jealousy to take possession of your breast. If you once admit this passion, it may terminate in your ruin. It will lead you to consider every seeming inattention, as a proof of his want of affection. You will conclude, *he is tired of his toy and is looking out for another*. This thought once admitted, will have an infatuating influence over your mind. Not only your actions will express your suspicion, but you will unguardedly speak it out, perhaps in terms of reproach.—Your good husband, stabbed to the very heart, may possibly with eyes full of tears clasp you in his arms and assure you of his love. But all will be vain, jealousy once admitted contaminates the soul. He will

scarcely turn his back, before the old impression will revive.

His tears and entreaties will be considered as evidence of his guilt, and you will wretchedly settle upon this conclusion. "*I am disagreeable, he is gone to carress the happy fair one whose company is preferred.*"

6. As you regard your own bliss, speedily check all thoughts of this kind, as soon as they arise in your mind. If indulged, they will have a baneful effect upon your temper, and spread a gloom over your countenance, so as to strip you of every charm. Your husband repelled from time to time, will at length become indifferent, and leaving you to languish in your distress, he will seek for amusement where it may be found. And thus you will bring upon yourself the very evil, against which you would make your mistaken defence.

7. If you have already proved the truth of these reflections by sad experience, I know you are ready to excuse yourself, because the whole proceeded from the most sincere affection. But you should consider that the anxiety and distress which are so often depicted in your countenance, might with equal propriety, lead your companion to doubt the sincerity of your love. And for any thing you know to the contrary, a suspicion of this

kind is at the bottom of the whole mischief. Do not act like stubborn children, rejecting that happiness which is entirely in your own power.

8. If he do not come in, the very hour or day that you expect him, instead of accusing him with neglect, be the considerate woman, and take into view the various and unavoidable delays with which he must meet in transacting his business. And be assured, for I speak from experience, that in many instances he sacrifices his most sincere wishes to be with you, for what he considers necessary for the present. He is bound to provide for you and your children. In easy circumstances there is most satisfaction, and he feels a strong desire to secure this foundation for your future happiness. Receive him then with gladness as often as he comes in, shew him that you are happy in his company, and let the preparations made for his reception, prove to him, that he holds a considerable share in your thoughts and affections when he is absent. Such conduct will endear you to his heart, and secure to you all the attention and regard you so ardently desire.

9. Do not suppose, that my plan implies that the husband has nothing to do. So far from this he is bound "To love and cherish his wife, as his own flesh." But I repeat it,

this obligation seems in a great degree, to rest on the condition of a loving and cheerful submission on the part of the wife. Here again perhaps you object and say, "Why not the husband, first shew a little condescension as well as the wife?" I answer for these plain reasons. It is not his disposition; it is not the custom but with the henpecked; it is not his duty; it is not implied in the marriage contract; it is not required by law or gospel.

10. I presume you are not one of those ladies who indulge a mean opinion of their companions, and are indeed ashamed of them. This can happen in no case where there is not a want of information and judgment. If you stooped in marrying him, do not indulge the thought, that you added to his respectability. Never tell him "you lifted him out of the ashes." For it will be hard for you to extricate yourself from this difficulty. "If you stooped of necessity, because you could get no one else, the obligation is on your own side. If you stooped of choice, who ought to be blamed but yourself? Besides it will be well to remember that when you became his wife, he became your head, and your supposed superiority was buried in that voluntary act.

CHAPTER III.

WIFE OUGHT NOT TO APPEAR IN THE HUSBAND'S BUSINESS.

There are women in the world, who arrogate to themselves, superior skill in the management of an estate, suppose they have great judgment in the value of property, and therefore wrest every thing out of the hands of their husbands, and convert the poor men into perfect cyphers. I hold the disposition and conduct of such women in great contempt, and I pity the *poor inoffensive creature of a man*, who can submit to be so degraded. *Yet it must be acknowledged, that where the man falls into the hands of a termagant*, he may find *it necessary to purchase peace on any terms.*

Men and women appear to best advantage each in their own proper station. Had it been my lot, to have taken one of those *man-like ladies*, whenever there happened to be company at my house, I should have made it my business, to brush the floor, rub the furniture, wash the tea equipage, scold the maids, talk about the kitchen and dairy, &c. and apologize as I procedeed, by giving intimation, that I had made an exchange of provinces with my good wife, by way of mutual accommodation.

Such conduct would at least shew, how aukwardly a man appears in acting the part of a woman, and of course would lead a woman of common sense to conclude, that she could not appear to much better advantage, when engaged in the capacity of a man.

If it were to save appearances only, the husband ought at least to *seem* to be the head. And therefore if you are determined to rule him, adopt the following plan. "When any article of property is to be bought or sold, take him aside, teach him the price to be given or received, point out the kind of payment, the time when to be paid, &c. &c. let the whole business be properly adjusted, and then let the poor fellow go forward and seem to act like a man." It is shocking to every man of sense, to see a woman interfere publicly, fly into a passion, and declare *point blank* the thing shall not be. Indeed if she had the true spirit of a woman, she would blush to acknowledge herself the wife of such a dastardly man as would submit to such treatment.

CHAPTER IV.

THE SURE WAY OF HAPPINESS IN THE MARRIED STATE.

The great point for securing happiness in the married state, is, to be mutually accommodating. The parties should look over one another's faults, and contemplate one another's excellencies. Nothing else will do.—We all have our defects, and it is much better to dwell on your own faults, than on those of your husband. For by so doing, you gradually correct yourself, to your own advantage. But if you pry deeply into his faults, you may make discoveries, which will serve only to lessen your esteem, and of course to detract from your happiness.

"A certain man bought a farm, and after a year or two, in conversation with his neighbour, he made heavy complaints how much he had been disappointed. Did you not see this land (says his neighbour) before you bought it? Oh yes, I saw it often. Do you not understand soils? I think I do tolerably. Did you not examine it with care? Not so much as I should have done. Standing at a certain place, it looked admirably, the fences were new and looked exceedingly neat, the house had been just painted a stone colour with panneling, the windows were large and elegant; but I neglected entirely, to examine the sufficiency of the materials, or the disposition of the apartments. There were in the month of April, two beautiful springs, but since I have lived here, they have been dry every year before the middle of June.—Did you not enquire of those who lived on the place of the permanence of the springs? No indeed I omitted it. Had you the full measure you were promised? Yes every acre. Was the right complete and valid? Yes, yes, perfectly good, no man in America can take it from me. Were you obliged to take it up in part of a bad debt? No, nothing like it. I took such a fancy for it all at once, that, I pestered the man from week to week to let me have it. Why really then, says his neighbour, I think you had better keep your complaints to yourself. Cursing and fretfulness will never turn stone into earth, or sand into loam; but I can assure you, that frugality, industry, and good culture, will make a bad farm very tolerable, and an indifferent one truly good."*

The application is easy, and you may occasionally read this story of the land purchaser to your husband; and if you will act

* Witherspoon

wisely, you will consider on either side, *that you are bound to be companions for life.*

How foolish it is to indulge in disputation and petty quarrels! Whoever may have been in fault, do not wait one for the other to shew marks of contrition. Let it rather be the emulation between you, who shall have the credit of making the first advances towards a reconciliation. After having slept in separate beds, and like two foolish children, refused to speak for a week or two, or more, you must at length make peace. Better then to do it immediately. It has been a rule with me for some years, that as often as any little jar may happen in my family, not a single night shall pass without a restoration of peace.

Do you so too, and some eight or ten years hence, you will thank me for the hint.

Should you be at a loss how to introduce the negociation of the peace, you might just say to each other, "let us remember the folly of Doctor Witherspoon's land purchaser."

CHAPTER V.

ONE WORD IN FAVOUR OF ECONOMY.

Strict adherence to the conduct recommended in the former chapters, is highly im portant. But I must inform you, that good economy and judicious house-wifery must also be added, or your happiness can by no means be complete. It affords a dismal prospect to a man who wishes to make a living, to find a double and tripple quantity of every article of family consumption necessary, to meet his wife's regulations and management.

Although happiness is not made up of wealth, yet a certain ease of circumstances contributes very much towards it. Hence it is, that "through all the lower or middle ranks of life, there is generally a good measure of matrimonial or domestic comfort, where their circumstances are easy, or their estate growing. Not only from their being freed from one of the most usual causes of peevishness and discontent, but also, because the affairs of a family are very seldom in a thriving state, unless *both* contribute their share of diligence ; so that they have not only a common happiness to share, but a joint merit in procuring their estate." Men may talk in raptures, and women may be puffed up with vain conceit, of youth, beauty, wit, sprightliness, and a hundred other shining qualities ! " but after seven years cohabitation, not one of them is to be compared, to good family management, which is seen at every meal, and felt every hour in the husband's purse.*

But as something more may be said of the duties of wives and husbands when I come to treat of the management of children, I shall proceed to consider some of the diseases, to which you may be subject in consequence of marriage.

CHAPTER VI.

SIGNS OF CONCEPTION, &c.

On various accounts it is considered necessary for married ladies to know when conception takes place. This point is not easily ascertained. Yet by proper observation most women may obtain a knowledge of it, sufficient to answer every necessary purpose. Many changes take place through the course of pregnancy; these I will state with the degree of certainty to be ascribed to them.

The breasts are commonly more or less affected. They are in some degree enlarged, and at the same time shooting pains are felt in them. As this enlargement advances the

* Witherspoon.

dark coloured ring which surrounds the nipple sometimes puts on a deeper hue.

Some unusual sensations will also be felt about the region of the womb. But neither of these marks are to be considered infallible and necessary, because there are frequent instances in which they do not occur at all.

Another appearance is the rising of the navel. The little cavity which this makes gradually fills up, so as to become an even surface. This is a pretty common and almost certain mark of pregnancy.

The stomach is affected with great sickness which is followed with vomiting and heartburn, loss of appetite and indigestion. This is a very general symptom.

The bowels do not escape the effects of this grand revolution. A considerable change from the usual condition commonly takes place. Those who have been habitually costive, will be troubled with a looseness, and those subject to diarrhea, will mostly become costive. But as these changes do also attend the times of menstruation they are not certain evidences of a state of pregnancy.

A feverish disposition attended with weakness and loss of flesh frequently affects those women who were before in pretty good health. But this is by no means universal, because there are some who fatten and become more healthy than at other times.

In some instances an universal fretfulness and impatience take place. If these tempers are not indulged in health, and befall you merely as symptoms of pregnancy your husband and friends will meet them with compassion. Resentment would indeed be cruel and unpardonable.

The head seldom escapes complaint, it is commonly so affected as to produce pain, giddiness, dimness of sight, sleepiness, and in some instances, though rarely, convulsion and palsy.

Sometimes a strange fluttering at the heart is felt which gives needless alarm as it implies no danger.

An entire suppression of the menses attends almost every case of pregnancy.* But as suppressions may be brought on by other causes this cannot be an infallible mark.

Difficult and even painful evacuations of the urine must not be omitted, because they frequently take place.

A peculiar loathing of animal food, and particularly of some favorite dish is one very common symptom.

Some new passion sometimes springs up.

---

*I have myself known exceptions.

This, whenever it happens, is a very certain mark. Doctor Rush in his lectures at the University of Pennsylvania gives an instance of one lady who feels a strange inclination to theft every time of her pregnancy.

At some time of gestation the child will move itself so strongly as to be felt by its mother. The first perception of this motion, is called the *quickening*. Most women suppose that this circumstance takes place at a certain and invariable stage of pregnancy.—But in fact it varies from the end of the tenth to the twenty-fifth week. The most common time however is about the sixteenth. At this time a few drops of blood pretty generally appear, without injury.

With the delicate in the first time of their pregnancy the *quickening* frequently excites considerable agitation with fainting and hysterics. For the fainting see part I. chap. IX.

CHAPTER VII.

THE PAINS ATTENDANT ON PREGNANCY PERHAPS NECESSARY.

Although the symptoms attendant on a state of pregnancy vary in different women, and although the same woman is seldom affected the same way with her different children, yet in almost every instance the case will be troublesome and distressing. But as the God of nature does nothing in vain, these distresses seem to be directed to an intended valuable end. For it is a fact that such of the ladies as are most subject to them do not often miscarry, and in the end fare better than those who escape. This consideration may afford you some consolation, when you meet with the common lot of your sex. I shall however distinctly re-consider the painful symptoms of gestation, and make known to you the conduct proper to be pursued, and the remedies to be employed when they occur.

CHAPTER VIII.

EXERCISE, DIET, &c.

It is a common opinion, that breeding women ought to live indolently and feast luxuriously as they are able, lest by exercise they should injure, or by abstinence debilitate the expected child. The conduct to which this opinion leads may happen to be proper. But it is possible it should be extremely wrong.—Those ladies who are accustomed to idleness and who of course cannot take any considerable degree of exercise without great consequent soreness or even fever, ought by no means to indulge in riding on horseback, running or romping, in any stage of pregnancy. Such too if of a full habit and feverish, ought not to take full meals nor too rich diet. It is worthy of remark, that, those who enjoy all the advantages of fortune, and who on this account are envied by the common people, are more subject to miscarriages and all the painful symptoms of gestation, than those who are under the necessity of labouring hard for a living. The poor man's house is filled with healthy children, while the rich with difficulty raises up an helpless heir, on whom to confer his estate and his diseases. The female slave is healthy and prolific, while the mistress is sickly and barren. Women of a full habit, when pregnant, ought to let blood at proper intervals. Some say particularly about the third and seventh month. It must be improper to fix upon any particular month for the purpose. But as often as pain and swimming of the head, giddiness and dimness of sight, pains in the loins and hips, with a sense of fulness of blood occur, six or eight ounces or more should be drawn from the arm. In the mean time she should avoid wine and spiritous liquors of every kind, rich sauces and flesh diet. Nature herself seems to favour this intention, by bringing about a loathing of food, and a due degree of abstinence will frequently prevent the necessity of blood-letting. Those who happen to be in a low state of health, and much emaciated about the time of conception, may find it necessary to take all the nourishment they can well bear, and at the same time to use friction of the flesh brush or flannel, with moderate exercise, for the improvement of their appetite and strength. Those who have been subject to obstructed or immoderate menses, attended with paleness, debility, and a disposition to bloat, may use wine, bark, steel, &c. with as much exercise as can be taken without fatigue. I met with a case in the year 1800, Mrs. F. W. who had six times miscarried from debility, and never had borne a living child. On application to me, I advised bark, steel, exercise, &c. the next pregnancy was nearly successful. The same plan was continued, and the eighth time of her gestation, she bore a fine girl, and her health was restored.

The happier class of women, who are in the habit of daily labour and continued exercise, may continue their engagements as before, except only, that it may be necessary to abate from their common fatigue, in a gradual manner, as they advance in pregnancy.—They should abstain from those things which are disagreeable, and eat moderately of such as are still pleasant; and in most instances little else will be wanting. If however, any of the symptoms threatening danger should present themselves, a little blood should be drawn from the arm, and repeated as often as necessary.

CHAPTER IX.

SICKNESS OF THE STOMACH AND VOMITING.

Great sickness of the stomach and vomiting are very common complaints in the early parts of pregnancy. In some instances the vomiting continues through the whole course of gestation, and in others disappears after some weeks, but to return again towards its close.

If the vomiting should happen only in the early part of the day and is not too violent, although an inconvenience it will seldom be injurious. Indeed it will generally prevent the necessity of employing a puke. But when the vomiting is violent in a case where there is full habit of body, it is often necessary to let blood from eight to ten ounces from the arm. After the bleeding, and in cases where through the weakness of the patient no blood can be spared, the vomiting may be removed by some of the following remedies.

1. Magnesia two teaspoonfuls in a cup of peppermint tea, to be repeated every one, two or three hours.

2. Salt of tartar 20 grains, lime juice or good vinegar half an ounce, spring water one and a half ounces, common syrrup a spoonful: to be speedily mixed together and taken while in a state of evervescence. It may be repeated once in three or four hours if necessary.

3. Or elixer vitrol, fifteen or twenty drops in a little water, or weak spirit and water made pleasant with sugar, to be repeated several times in the day.

4. Or an infusion of columbo or camomile with orange peel in boiling water. The columbo is thought most effectual. It may be so managed, as to take from ten to twenty grains, for every two or three hours if necessary.

5. Or where the vomiting is excessive, opium from half a grain to a grain, to be re-

peated every one or two hours till the complaint abates.*

6. Or in many instances a cloth folded so as to be four inches square, and moistened with the tincture of opium, and applied externally to the region of the stomach, gives great relief.

7. Where there is great and distressing efforts to vomit, without any evacuation, it will be proper to make use of small doses of ipecacuanha, from ten to twenty grains according to circumstances, and to be repeated as often as it may be found necessary. There is no kind of danger in administering a gentle puke to a pregnant woman.

8. A change of posture, whether from lying down to sitting up, or the contrary, ought to be brought about in a very gradual manner. Simple as this direction may appear, it will be attended with considerable benefit.

9. Some find relief from the sickness of the stomach by chewing fresh, hard well made, water biscuit ; sucking limes ; lying much of their time in bed ; taking fresh air ; riding out on a pleasant gaited horse, or in a carriage ; eating at such times, and so often

* Where there is fever, opium is improper without some previous evacuation. In most cases blood-letting should be premised

as to avoid an empty stomach, whether day or night: And for this purpose some have used gingerbread with advantage.

CHAPTER X.

HEART BURN.

Breeding women are also frequently subject to a painful sense of heat in the throat, with belching of a hot and sour liquid, which is very distressing. This affection is commonly called heart burn. If the complaint be violent, nothing perhaps is better than a small dose of ipecacuanha, so as to procure a motion or two. After the puke use the following preparation.

Magnesia and spirits of sal ammoniac, or spirits of heartshorn, of each the eighth of an ounce; cinnamon water, or a strong infusion of cinnamon, three eighths of an ounce; pure spring water five ounces. Of this, two or three table spoonfuls to the dose, as often as the heart-burn is distressing. If however, this complaint is the consequence of a loss of digestive power, the strength of the stomach must be restored by the use of some bitter infusion, as orange peel, camomile, columbo, bark, &c. Some preparation

one

of steel, with exercise, might also be employed.

CHAPTER XI.

COSTIVENESS.

Great costiveness frequently attends the advanced stages of pregnancy, and in many instances passes unnoticed without any considerable injury. Where it is found necessary, the bowels may be kept gently open by the help of a little manna, magnesia, senna, castoroil, the purging salts, or Lee's pills.—But any of the other articles may be prefered before the pills, if they can be conveniently obtained.

There is one species of this complaint, occasioned by a collection of hardened feces in the lower part of the intestines. This sometimes requires the use of an instrument, somewhat in the form of a scoop, to break the clod. When broken, it may be washed away with repeated glysters.

CHAPTER XII.

TOOTH-ACHE.

Tooth-ache is a very distressing symptom, and may be removed by applying small blisters behind the ears, or repeated doses of opium, or finally by having the defective tooth drawn out. If however, it be the consequence of fever, blood-letting may be necessary. And if it should take place at the same time with a sicknesss of the stomach, a puke will most likely afford relief.

CHAPTER XIII.

PILES.

Most fleshy women, and more commonly those who lead sedentary lives, are subject to the distressing complaint called the *piles*.—Such too as are much troubled with costiveness, seldom escape this disorder. By whatever means the disposition to the piles is formed, it generally is more troublesome in the last months of pregnancy, than at other times. If the attack be of the more moderate kind, a gentle dose of cream of tartar and flowers of sulphur combined, will afford considerable relief. Cold applications of any kind, as of cloth wetted in cold water, or spirit and water, would answer the purpose. Also the following ointment. Take the yolk of one egg, tincture of opium or laudanum three tea spoonfuls, neatsfoot or other oil one table spoonful, to be mixed and applied.—Let the tincture and the yolk of the egg be first mixed together, and afterwards the oil may be added. This ointment gives relief when much disposed to itch. If they protrude outwards, press them between the thumb and finger and at the same time anoint and put them up carefully. Those subject to this complaint ought to lie down upon their backs for a few minutes after every stool. I have known this precaution to do much towards preventing their return when once removed. I am told an ointment made of the oak ball, powdered and stewed in hogs lard, is a valuable remedy, and there is no reason to doubt its efficacy.*

CHAPTER XIV.

DIARRHEA.

This complaint is sometimes very troublesome and injurious to pregnant women. If attended with fever, let blood from the arm from six to ten or fifteen ounces according to

* Take one inch of a tallow candle, round its corners and smear it well on all sides with mercurial ointment. Put this up the rectum on going to bed, and let it remain till morning.

the strength of the patient. Should there be much sickness at the stomach, a puke is advisable. For this purpose, take from ten to twenty or thirty grains of ipecacuanha. After the bleeding, or puke, or both when necessary, it may be advantageous to use a portion of rhubarb and calomel. Rhubarb, fifteen or twenty grains ; calomel, from three to five grains. This last is necessary, where there is irregularity in the secretion of the bile.

When the necessary evacuations are procured, take gum opium, twelve grains ; powdered rhubarb, forty-eight grains ; ipecacuanha, twelve grains ; syrrup, as much as is sufficient to make them into pills. The whole to form twenty-four pills, one of which may be given every six or eight hours. In the mean time, the starch glyster with tincture of opium, or a glyster made with boiled flour, or of mutton broth with the same tincture, may be thrown up every three or four hours if necessary. Sometimes blistering the wrists and ankles is found beneficial after the feverish sypmtoms are subdued. Bathing the feet frequently in hot water, might also be tried.

CHAPTER XV

STRANGURY.

A frequent inclination to void the urine, which is discharged in small quantities with painful sensations at every evacuation. This complaint is called *Strangury.* The long retention of the urine so often practised by the ladies from delicacy, frequently brings it on. But the pressure of the enlarged womb upon the bladder, is the cause of it in the last months of pregnancy. If there be fever, let blood from the arm. Give frequent glysters of warm milk and water. Manna half an ounce, and sweet oil one ounce, may be given as a gentle purge. Frequent doses of purified salt petre may be taken in mallows tea. Or spirits of nitre forty drops, may be taken in a drink of barley water, every two hours. Two grains of opium may sometimes be taken, and warm wet cloths may be applied to the belly and groins, to be renewed as often as they begin to grow cool.

If a total suppression takes place, send for a physician who can introduce an instrument for the purpose of drawing off the water.* It may not be amiss to add here, that sometimes an incontinence of urine attends in the

* This instrument is called a Catheter.

latter stages of pregnancy. For relief in this case, use occasionally, gentle purges, avoid sudden exertion, and spend more of your time in bed. But whenever this complaint occurs it is one very sure indication that the child is rightly presented for the birth.

CHAPTER XVI.

FLUOR ALBUS.

For a description and the cure of this complaint see chapter XXIII. part I. It seldom does any injury, and is commonly followed by an easy delivery. Where it becomes very profuse, and where it violently attacks those subject to miscarriage, recourse may be had to the proper remedies, and especially to the injection agreeable to the above reference. If attended with heat and fever, moderate blood-letting and gentle purges should be occasionally repeated.

CHAPTER XVII.

VARICOUS SWELLINGS OF THE LEGS.

Sometimes a strange distention of the viens of the legs takes place in the last months of gestation. To those who may never have seen such a case, it might give considerable alarm; but it is not followed by any immediate danger; a disagreeable numbness commonly attends it, and the distorted veins elevate the skin, producing great unevenness. The proper remedies here are small frequent blood-letting and gentle purging.

CHAPTER XVIII.

CRAMP

Is another complaint which occurs chiefly during the last months. For the cure keep the bowels gently open. If it attend a full habit, bleed. If it should come on in the night, jump out of the bed and stand upon the feet till it goes off. Sometimes to grasp a cane or bed post or a roll of sulphur in the hand, affords relief.

CHAPTER XIX.

INQUIETUDE OR WANT OF SLEEP.

A peculiar kind of restlessness sometimes takes place, which is attended with pain in the region of the womb. This pain is most severe at night, and resembles labour pains. It frequently prevails against a strong inclination to sleep. When in this situation the patient frequently feels the want of cool air. But after all her perplexity she will find herself refreshed by the morning.

For the cure in this case also, small bleedings and gentle laxatives. Or take a drink of cold water on lying down. Also one end of a wetted towel might be wrapped round one hand, and the other end be let to hang out of the bed. This last is a simple and pleasant remedy.

CHAPTER XX.

FEAR OF DEATH.

A distressing fear of the event of parturition, sometimes takes possession of pregnant women, as the dreaded time approaches.— Such should be taught reliance on the protection of *Providence*. If however this dread be attended with increased heat, a white scurf on the tongue, quick pulse, and especially if there be a fixed pain in the belly, there is certainly a fever present, which ought by no means to be neglected. It requires blood-letting, and frequently a repetition of it with gentle purges. Thirty or forty drops of the spirits of nitre may then be given in some kind of drink. Every kind of exercise must for the time be avoided, and a light diet only should be taken. If these things should be neglected through inattention, or want of the necessary means, the dread of death may be realized, and then her friends may condemn themselves in vain, for having treated a serious complaint with levity.

CHAPTER XXI.

DROPSICAL SWELLINGS, &c.

Dropsical swellings of the lower extremities often occur, and sometimes extend up to the sides of the lower belly. In some instances, the external parts of generation are distended to such a degree as to be very painful, and to make it difficult for the patent to walk. This swelling peculiar to a state of pregnancy, has been sometimes mistaken for common dropsy, and has led to the use of improper medicines, and even to the operation of tapping, bringing about the death of mother and child, to the disgrace of the science of medicine. In this case also, small bleedings and gentle purges, repeated as occasion may require, are the most safe and proper remedies.

CHAPTER XXII.

DISTENTION OF THE ABDOMEN.

The belly is sometimes so stretched as to crack the skin, afterwards forming scars of a peculiar kind. For ease and safety in such a case, let the skin be anointed with mutton suet beat up with a strong decoction of red roses. When the swelling hangs so low, as to be troublesome and painful, relief may be had by passing a broad bandage under it, to be supported by a soft and springy strap of some kind, passed over the shoulders. This aid would be particularly advantageous, to such as are under the necessity of walking about. Sometimes a rupture of the navel is the consequence of this great distention ; but this will be readily removed after the birth of the child, by the aid of simple pressure only.

CHAPTER XXIII.

MOLES, &c.

By whatever cause the womb is sufficiently distended, all the symptoms attending pregnancy in its natural state, may be excited.—This distention is sometimes the consequence of dropsy of a particular kind, as of small vessicles of water hung together in the form of clusters; sometimes it follows imperfect conception, in which case a monster or shapeless mass is produced; and sometimes it is the consequence of *moles* so called.—These are nothing more than a collection of the thicker parts of the blood, and happen sometimes to women subject to immoderate menses; but chiefly take place after a miscarriage. The monsters have their cake and cord, but moles have neither.

CHAPTER XXIV.

ABORTION.

The instructions given chap. VIII. part II. are particularly intended to guard against abortion. In addition to those remarks, I must here add, that this event is but seldom the effect of any kind of moderate exertion. And, although it may have been ascribed to a great variety of accidents, yet in most cases, it is the consequence of some disease of the mother or child. It will therefore be prudent, in all cases where there is a repetition of miscarriage, to obtain the advice of some judicious physician. For if any particular disease or constitutional defect on the part of the parent be the cause, all common attempts for her relief will probably fail.

The symptoms which indicate the approach of this misfortune are various. "But there is generally pain in the back, belly and inferior extremities, that is, the thighs, legs, &c." with a sense of weight and weakness in the region of the womb, frequent inclination to void the urine, with a continual painful urging to go to stool. But the most certain sign of an abortion, is a discharge of blood, and this is the most dangerous and alarming appearance. Various methods have been adopted for moderating and staying it, see chap. XXI. part I.

But perhaps the most effectual of any is the application of a cloth wetted with vinegar and water, which should be applied over the parts, and so firmly pressed with the hand, as instantly to retard, or stop the stream of blood. Where there are irregular pains without much fever, small doses of opium frequently repeated, may be of service. If fever be present, then instead of the opium, small doses of ipecacuanha would be preferable. When violent floodings take place in the advanced stages of pregnancy, so that it may be difficult to determine, whether the case is an abortion or premature labour, it has been advised to proceed immediately to deliver the woman. But it scarcely ever is necessary to afford assistance by hand. If however it should seem not safe, to depend on the usual remedies, it might be proper to break the membranes, and discharge the waters. But even this should be attempted with the greatest caution. For says Doctor Denman, "In abortions, dreadful and alarming as they are sometimes, it is great comfort to know, that they are almost universally void of danger either from the hemorrage, or on any other account." A case may occur however, where it becomes necessary to deliver the woman by art, in order to save her from perishing by mere loss of blood. When this is suspected procure the aid of the most skillful physician or midwife, See part III. chap. XXI. XXII, &c. &c.

☞ To prevent miscarriage and at the same time to secure an easy and safe delivery, every pregnant lady who can bear it, is hereby most earnestly requested, to make a very frequent use of laxative medicines thro' the whole course, and particularly through the last months of pregnancy.—Castor oil—manna—sweet oil—decoction of elder roots, or the like—any of these will answer, but perhaps the oils ought to be preferred in almost every case.

END OF THE SECOND PART.

Part Third.

Hints for the Midwife.

CHAPTER I.

INTRODUCTION.

WHEN it is granted that there are some women skilled in the art of *Midwifery*, the known liberality of the ladies will indulge me in a declaration that most of those who make pretensions to this important profession are exceedingly ignorant and self-conceited. A great proportion of them have been introduced into the practice by being *caught* as they commonly call it, with some one or more women. Their known ignorance forbade them to be officious, and nature unassisted, or rather *uninterrupted*, performed her own office properly. The success in each case unjustly attributed to the attending woman, encouraging others to employ her, she is presently considered a deep proficient in the art. Her vanity keeps an equal pace with the fame of her skill, and in a little time she affects considerable knowledge of most diseases, is dubbed a mighty doctress, and not unfrequently has the address to impose her fanciful prescriptions upon a whole extensive neighborhood.

I have no wish that all such should be forsaken by no means ; expediency and their popularity forbid. But it is right to demand of them a submission to their own proper station, for as often as they exceed their due bounds they do violence to the laws of God and the cause of humanity. Within the limits of a certain sphere, they might be useful and respectable. If they would extend their usefulness, let them first learn how little knowledge they possess, that they may exert themselves in making more extensive attainments.*

There is no doubt that all wish their services to be beneficial or that many are reluctantly drawn into the practice. But however good or humane their intention, instances of irretreivable mischief have occurred

* I have no intention of calling in question the capacity of the ladies for understanding this or any other art or science. It is my candid opinion that, female genius with equal cultivation would excel that of the males.

from their ignorance and ill-timed officiousness. To the candid and humane, the following hints will therefore be acceptable.

CHAPTER II.

NECESSARY DEFINITIONS.

As I shall be under the necessity of using names of parts not commonly understood, I shall state them with their definitions as far as necessary for my present design.

1. The *abdomen*, is the name given to the belly. It is the soft covering of the bowels, extending from the breast down to the following bone, which is called,

2. The *pubis*, this bone stands forwards, forming an arch between the hips and is called by some the *bearing bone*. It has a peculiar kind of joint in the middle, which sometimes opens in cases of difficult labour; and when this happens it is commonly followed by a collection of matter, distressing to the last degree, very difficult to cure and sometimes fatal to the patient.

3. The *Sacrum* is that part of the bones which is fixed between the hips backwards, and is opposite to the *pubis*. The sacrum extends itself downwards and forwards form-

ing a curve and makes it necessary to regulate the passage of the child in a corresponding direction.

4. The large passage or cavity made by these two bones together with the other bones of the hips is called the *pelvis*. If this cavity is much less than common, or out of shape, so as to prevent the passage of the child, the pelvis is said to be distorted. This distortion may be effected several ways. The common distance between the sacrum and pubis is rather more than four inches; but it is sometimes found to be no more than one.—The lower part of the sacrum which bends forwards and inwards forming a curve as above, in young women admits of a little motion backwards so as to make the passage of the child more easy. But in some instances, especially in those women who do not marry till they become old maids, it is so strong as not to admit of any motion at all.—In addition to this it sometimes bends so far inwards as very much to obstruct the passage.

5. The *mons veneris*, is the fatty substance which covers the pubis and extends downwards and sideways towards the two groins.

6. The *Labia*, the two thick soft pieces of skin which pass on either side, still downwards from the mons veneris.

7. The *pudendum*, external parts of generation, of these the labia are the principal parts.

8. The *perinaeum*, the part which begins at the lower angle of the *labia* and extends backwards to the *anus* or fundament. This part is subject to be torn in child-bearing.

9. The *vagina*, the passage from the pudendum to the womb.

10. The *uterus* the name of the womb.

11. At the upper end of the *vagina* is an opening into the womb called the *os uteri* or mouth of the womb.

12. The *placenta*, the afterbirth, called also *the cake*, and with the membranes including the child waters, &c. is sometimes called the *secundines*.

13. The *umbilical cord*, the navel string.

14. The *foetus*, the child while in the womb. To these names I will add in this place the five following terms expressive of certain changes which take place in the act of child-bearing.*

---

*I am informed that some of my fair readers are a good deal exasperated with me for exposing "*female weakness*." I am extremely sorry for their want of information and judgment Is not such knowledge as I have made public necessary for female safety? Certainly it is. How then in the name of common sense could it ever be made sufficiently known without such *exposure*, if they will have it by that name? Strange

15. *Parturition*, the act of bringing forth a child. It is another name for *labour*.

16. *Dilatation*, the act of stretching and opening at the same time. This is applied to the os uteri and to the pudendum.

17. *Distension*, the act of stretching or making more open.

18. *Expell*, the act of turning out; this is performed by the uterus when it contracts, which it endeavors to do by certain periodical exertions called *pains*.

19. *Presentation*, the act of presenting.—This term is applied to the position of the child, and particularly to the part of the child which is first sensible to the touch, at the mouth of the womb, when labour is coming on.

CHAPTER III.

NATURAL POSITION, PRESENTATION, &c.

It was formerly believed that the child in the natural position in the uterus was sitting with its face towards the abdomen, and that towards the time of parturition, by the weight

indeed that *female delicacy* should demand a sacrifice of thousands of the best of women, and tens of thousands of tender innocents, to keep it in countenance! Truth is invincible, and time will unfold its power.

of its head, it revolved itself and turned its head downward, ready to pass through the pelvis. This change was called *presenting to the birth.* But more accurate observations have proved this opinion to be false. No such revolution is necessary. And unless some circumstance has occurred to change the position of the child, it is always proper for the presentation If therefore the presentation be a natural one, the head is downward resting upon the pubis, One side of the head is towards the abdomen and the other towards the sacrum, or in some degree obliquely varying from this position. The bulk of the body is commonly on the right side and the limbs are turned towards the left.

CHAPTER IV.

DEFINITION OF LABOUR, &c.

The common time for complete gestation is forty weeks, at the expiration of which, the process of labour commences.

This process is not the effect of any particular exertion of the child. Nor of any united efforts of the mother and child. But it is a peculiar power of the womb itself, by which at the time appointed by the God of nature, it endeavours to expel its contents.

Labours are either *natural*, *difficult*, *preternatural* or *complex*.

1. Every labour should be called *natural* if the head of the child present; if the labour be compleated within twenty-four hours, and if no artificial aid be required.

2. If the labour be prolonged beyond twenty-four hours, it may be called *difficult*.

3. If any other part except the head present, the labour may be said to be *preternatural*.

4. All other cases requiring aid, may be said to be *complex*.

CHAPTER V.

SYMPTOMS OF PRESENT LABOUR.

The first symptom of present labour is anxiety, arising from a dread of danger or doubt of safety. This anxiety will be increased, if the patient should have heard of accidents or deaths in any late similar case. It is the duty of the midwife to soothe and comfort her when in this situation, by suitable language, and a diligent and proper attention to every complaint. But in the mean time, she should by no means be persuaded to offer assistance before it is necessary.

2. At the commencement of labour, women commonly have one or more chills, or fits of shivering, with or without a sense of cold. But should there be one strong and distinct chill or shivering fit, it may be a dangerous symptom.

3. There will be some difficulty in voiding the urine. It should therefore be evacuated frequently, otherwise it may ultimately become necessary to introduce a catheter.

4. There will sometimes be a frequent painful disposition to go to stool. This ought to be considered a favourable symptom. A glyster or two, prepared of milk and water or thin gruel, may serve to correct the pain. Or if no such disposition be present, the glysters may serve to evacuate the bowels artificially.

5. The mucous discharge, which before was without colour, after the commencement of labour will be tinged with blood. This appearance is commonly called the *shew*.

6. If together with the above symptoms the usual pains be present, the presumption is very strongly in favour of approaching parturition.

CHAPTER VI.

COMMON APPEARANCE OF TRUE PAINS.

1. The *true pains* usually begin in the loins or lower part of the back, pass round into the *abdomen*, and end at the pubis, or upper part of the thighs. Sometimes however they take the opposite direction, that is, beginning at the thighs or pubis, and ending in the loins. Sometimes too, they are confined to one particular spot, as the *back*, *abdomen*, *thighs*, and even to the knees, heels or feet; and in some instances, other parts are affected, as the stomach, head, &c.

2. The true labour pain is periodical, with intervals of twenty, fifteen, ten or five minutes, *and moderate pains frequently repeated are safer than more severe ones at greater intervals.*

3. An experienced midwife, may generally judge of the nature of present pains from the tone of the patient's voice. The first change effected by the pains, consists in a dilation of the parts. Forcible and quick distension, gives a sensation like that produced by the infliction of a wound, and the tone of voice will be in a similar manner interrupted and shrill. These are vulgarly called *cutting*, *grinding*, or *rending* pains. When the

internal parts are sufficiently opened, the child begins to descend, and then the patient is by her feelings obliged to make an effort to expel, and the expression will be made with a continued and grave tone of voice, or she will hold her breath and be silent. These are called *bearing pains*.

It is a common thing to say, that women have fruitless or unprofitable pain. This is an unfair and discouraging statement. No person in labour ever had a pain depending on her labour, which was in vain.

4. In the beginning the pains are usually slight in their degree, and have long intervals, but as the labour advances, they become more violent, and the intervals are shorter. Sometimes the pains are alternately, one stronger the next weaker, or one stronger and two weaker. But every variety has its own peculiar advantages, being wisely adapted to the state of the patient. Nothing therefore can be more preposterous, than any kind of artificial attempt to add to the strength of the pains, or to hasten their return. It is wrong even to direct the patient to *help herself. The supposed skill of midwives in these points, has done more mischief to society, than the most skillful practice ever did good.*

CHAPTER VII.

HOW FALSE PAINS MAY BE DETECTED AND REMOVED.

A case may occur, where it may be necessary to determine whether present pains be true or false; because if false pains be encouraged, or permitted to continue, they may at length occasion premature labour.

First then, some known cause commonly goes before and brings on false pains; as fatigue of any kind, especially too long standing on the feet, sudden and violent motion of the body, great costiveness, a diarrhea, a general feverish disposition, some violent agitation of the mind or the like.

2. But the most certain way for detecting false pains, is by an actual examination. This operation is commonly called *taking a pain.* The position in which women are placed, when it is thought necessary to examine them, varies in different countries, and indeed almost every midwife has her own opinion. But most *regular men*, direct the woman to repose on a couch or bed, upon her left side, with her knees bent and drawn up towards the abdomen. *And this is certainly the most convenient and decent method.* The examination should be performed with the utmost

care, decency and tenderness. If there be perceptible pressure on the *os uteri*, or if it be perceived to dilate during the continuance of a pain, the woman may be considered as really in labour. But if neither pressure nor dilatation can be felt, the conclusion may be drawn that the pains are false.

3. If it be determined, that the pains are false, it will be proper to attempt to remove them. When occasioned by fatigue of any kind, the patient should rest in bed. If she be of a feverish disposition, she should loose some blood. Generally it will be proper to give a dose or two of manna with sweet oil, or of castor oil or the like. Mild and opening glysters should be injected every three or four hours, till the bowels are emptied. After these evacuations, which should be repeated according to the exigency of the case, she should have half a grain of opium with one grain of ipecacuanha, every three hours till she is composed.

4. Let it be observed however, that an examination should never be made in too great haste. And if it be probable, that the patient is really in labour, an examination for determining the state of the presentation, ought not to be made until the membranes are broken, or till the *os uteri* is fully dilated. But more of this in another place.

CHAPTER VIII.

PROGRESS OF A NATURAL LABOUR.

There may be said to be three stages in the process of natural labour.

The *first* includes all the circumstances and changes which take place from the commencement of the pains, to the complete dilatation of the *os uteri*, the breaking of the membranes and the discharge of the waters.

The *second* includes those which occur, from the time of the opening of the *os uteri*, to the expulsion of the child.

And the *third* includes all the circumstances which relate to the separation and exclusion of the *placenta;* but to treat of each of these stages more particularly and in order.

1. The *os uteri* is not always found in the same central position, nor does it always dilate in the same length of time.

The first part of the dilatation is generally made very slowly, but when the membranes containing the waters begin to insinuate themselves, they act like a wedge, and the operation proceeds much more rapidly.

It cannot well be told with certainty how long time will be required in any case, for the complete dilatation of the *os uteri*, yet some conjecture may be made. If for example, after the pains have continued three hours, the *os uteri* should be dilated to the size of one inch, then two hours will be required for dilating it to two inches, and three more hours will be required for a complete dilatation; making in all eight hours. This calculation supposes the labour to go on regularly and with equal strength. But the *os uteri* sometimes remains for hours in the same state, and yet when it begins to dilate, the complete dilatation is soon perfected. Again, in some cases the dilatation proceeds on regularly for a while, and then is suspended for many hours, and afterwards returns with great vigour.

With first children, this stage is commonly tedious and very painful. Some considerable judgment is therefore necessary on the part of the midwife, for supporting the patience and confidence of the suffering woman. As the labour proceeds, the pains become more frequent and forcible. And if the dilatation should take place with difficulty, there will sometimes be a sickness of the stomach and vomiting. This is a favourable circumstance, and it commonly has a tendency to relax the system.

At length after a greater or lesser number of hours, as the case may be, the dilatation is effected. *But let it be carefully observed, that no artificial aid is to be offered during this part of the process.* It may indeed be well enough to pretend to assist, with the intention to compose the mind of the patient, and inspire her with confidence. *But be assured, that all manual interposition, will retard the progress of the dilatation.*

Let the patient and bye-stander be importunate. Pain on the one hand, and ignorance on the other may excuse them. But the midwife must be firm in the discharge of her duty.

Care must be taken, not to break the membranes should an examination be deemed necessary. When the *os uteri* is fully dilated, they are usually broken by the force of the pains. If this should not be the case, they will be protruded outwards, in the form of a bag, and then are of no further use. If the labour has not been disturbed, the child is commonly born speedily after the natural rupture of the membranes; and therefore if the birth be delayed after this event takes place, it will be a very proper time, to make a careful examination of the state of things.

Here I must be permitted to remark, that touching the parts too frequently is highly pernicious. The juices furnished by nature for moistening, softening and by these means preparing the parts for distention, must be improperly exhausted by repeated application of the hand. If the passage be thus left dry it will be much disposed to irritation, and the whole process may be deranged. In every difficult case which has come under my observation, I have been able to trace all the existing evils back, to the common error of too early *taking in hand*, as the operation is commonly called. Your pomatums, oils, lard, and ointments, are poor substitutes for natural fluids which are wiped away. Indeed they may do injury, by clogging the mouths of the little vessels through which those fluids are secreted. By escaping any such injury, it happens pretty commonly that women *taken at surprise*, have *better times* than when aided by the good midwife of the neighbourhood.

If there be no irregularity, nature is always competent to the task appointed her of God, and the only circumstances which can make it necessary to call in a midwife at all, are the *possibility of such irregularity* and the convenience of having her dexterity in management of the placenta, dressing the child, &c.

CHAPTER IX.

SECOND STAGE OF NATURAL LABOUR.

The second stage of labour includes all the circumstances attending the descent of the child through the pelvis, the dilatation of the external parts, and the final expulsion of the child. In general it will follow that the further the labour is advanced before the discharge of the waters, the more speedily and safely this second stage will be accomplished.

As the head of the child passes through the pelvis, it undergoes various changes of position, by which it is adapted to the form of each part of the passage; and that more or less readily according to the size of the head, strenth of the pains &c. And whether these changes are produced quickly, or in a tedious manner, whether in one or many hours, it can by no means be proper to interfere. For the powers of the constitution will produce their proper effect, with less injury and more propriety than the most dexterous midwife.

When the head begins to press upon the external parts; at first every pain may be suffered to have its full and natural effect. But when a part of the head is fully exposed, and the fore part of the perinæum is on the stretch, it is necessary to use some precaution to prevent its being torn; and the more expeditious the labour, the more is this caution necessary.

Some have thought, that if the external parts be very rigid, they should be frequently anointed with some kind of ointment. Nothing can equal the natural juices. But if from any cause the parts become heated and dry, flannels wrung out of warm water should be applied for some time, and afterwards some very mild ointment might not be amiss. Women with first children are most subject to inconvenience and difficulty in these respects.

To prevent any injury from lesion the external parts, the only safe and effectual plan is to retard for a certain time the passage of the head through them. Therefore, instead of encouraging the patient at this time, to use her utmost exertion to hasten the birth, she should be convinced of its impropriety, and be dissuaded from using any voluntary exertion. If she cannot be regulated according to your wishes, her efforts must be counteracted by some equivalent external resistance. This may be performed by placing the finger and thumb of the right hand upon the head of the child, during the time of a pain; or by placing the balls of one or both thumbs, on the thin edge of the perinæum. With first children, if there be great exertion, and much danger of a laceration, the right hand may be used as before, and the palm of the left hand wound round with a soft cloth, may be applied over the whole perinaeum, where it must be firmly continued during the violence of the pain. It is proper to proceed in this way, till the parts are sufficiently dilated. Then the head may be permitted to slide through them in the slowest and gentlest manner, paying the strictest attention till it is perfectly cleared of the perinaeum. If there should be any delay or difficulty, when the perinaeum slides over the face, the fore finger of the right hand, may be passed under its edge, by which it may be cleared of the mouth and chin, before the support given by the left hand be withdrawn.

The assistance should be applied in a proper direction, and with uniformity. The danger of injury to the external parts will be encreased by irregular or partial pressure.

The head being expelled, it is commonly deemed necessary to extract the body of the child without delay. But experience has now taught, that there is no danger, and that it is far safer for the mother and child, to wait for the return of the pains. And when the shoulders of the child begin to advance, and the external parts are again brought to the stretch, the same support should be given to the perinaeum as before. The child should then be conducted in a proper direction, so as to keep its weight from resting too heavily on the perinaeum. *Two or three pains are sometimes necessary for the expulsion of the shoulders after the head is born.*

The child should be placed in such a situation, that the external air may have free access to its mouth, but let its head be covered. Having taken the proper care of the mother, it will be necessary to proceed to the third and last part of the operation.

CHAPTER X.

THIRD STAGE OF NATURAL LABOUR, THE MANAGEMENT OF PLACENTA, &c.

There is a proper time for dividing the *funis* or umbilical cord. Before the child breathes and cries, a motion of the arteries of the cord may be felt beating like the pulse. But after it has breathed and cried, this pulsation or motion ceases, and the string becomes quite relaxed and soft. These circumstances ought to take place before the umbilical cord is divided. Ten, fifteen, and sometimes twenty minutes are required for the complete relaxation of the navel string. Then let it be tied in two places, and divide between them.

Soon after the birth of the child, the midwife should apply her hand upon the abdomen of the mother to determine whether there be another child, and whether the womb contracts in a manner favorable to the separation and removal of the cake.

Most women are extremely uneasy till the placenta is removed, and suppose the sooner it is accomplished the better; but this uneasiness is unnecessary, and all hurry is improper.

After the birth of the child let the first attention be paid to the mother. Tranquility should be restored to her mind, and the hurried circulation of the blood should be calmed. She should be recovered from her fatigue, and her natural state regained as soon as possible. With this design let her be kept quiet, affording her at the same time some suitable refreshment.

In the course of ten, fifteen or twenty minutes, the pains will return, for the purpose of expelling the placenta; and it will generally be expelled without any kind of artificial aid, which should never be employed where it can be avoided. But if it descend too slowly, the midwife may take hold of the cord and by pulling in a gentle manner and in a proper direction, may afford some assistance ; and this should be done only in time of a pain.

After the cake is brought down into the vagina, whether by the natural pains, or with the artificial aid as above, it must be suffered to remain there till excluded by the pains. This may prevent a dangerous flooding. If an hour be requisite for the exclusion, after it enters the vagina, no assistance ought to be offered, but after that time, it may again be gently pulled in the time of the pains. No objections should be raised to this plan from any supposed advantage to be derived to the child from laying the cake upon its belly, upon hot embers, in hot wine, or the like. All this is perfect folly.

Let it then be a settled point, that hurry is improper either in dividing the string, or removing the cake. Haste in the first may destroy the child, in the last must injure the mother in a greater or lesser degree. If the ill effects be not immediately perceived, she will at length be sensible of the injury, when her health gradually declines.

The conclusion to be drawn from the foregoing is, that parturition is a natural process of the constitution, which generally needs no assistance. And when it is natural it should always be suffered to have its own course without interruption.

CHAPTER XI.

INTRODUCTION TO DIFFICULT LABOURS.

In consequence of their natural construction, the women must be subject to great pain and difficulty in parturition; yet by the peculiar form of the mother, and the original construction of the head of the child, ample provision is made for overcoming all the difficulties to which they are subject. But by the customs of society, and various other causes, women are rendered subject to diseases and accidents which encrease their natural inconveniences, and produce new causes of danger. Therefore, there will be occasions which will require assistance.

The first distinction of labour, requiring the assistance of art, may be called *difficult* and every labour in which the head of the child presents, but which is delayed longer than twenty-four hours, ought to be classed under this head.

Difficult or tedious labours may be of four kinds.

I. Those which are rendered difficult from a too weak or an irregular action of the womb.

II. Those which are occasioned by a certain rigidity, or firmness of the parts, in consequence of which the dilatation is tedious and difficult.

III. Those in which a quick and easy passage of the head of the child is prevented, by some distortion of the pelvis, or too large a size of the head.

IV. Those which are rendered difficult from diseases of the soft parts.

CHAPTER XII.

FIRST KIND OF DIFFICULT LABOURS.

1. The action of the womb is sometimes too weak in consequence of great distention. In a case of this sort the safest, and frequently the only remedy, is to allow the patient sufficient time. In the mean time, she may be suffered to walk, or stand, pursue any amusement, or choose that position which she may prefer. Sometimes however frequent glysters of warm milk and water, or thin gruel might be injected. Or if the pains should be feeble, an come on in a ve-

ry slow manner, and if the labour be far advanced, it will be proper to give a glyster of gruel made more irritating by the addition of an ounce of common table salt, or a like quantity of purging salt; which ever may be most convenient.

2. The action of the womb may be feeble and tedious in consequence of being partial or incomplete. In a case of this kind, the patient will complain that the child lies very high in the stomach, or she will have cramp-like pains in various parts of the abdomen, which seem quite ineffectual. If these pains be great, and different from common *abour pains*, they are commonly the effect of a feverish disposition; and if so, the patient may loose small quantities of blood. She may take thirty or forty drops of spirits of nitre, in a cup of some kind of cooling tea, every two or three hours. Her bowels must be kept open with glysters, or gentle doses of manna, castor oil or purging salt; and sometimes it will be found useful to anoint the whole abdomen with warm oil. If little or no fever be present, she might walk about the room, in the intervals between the pains. If she should have suffered much and a long time, after the blood letting and a glyster or two, she should take forty-five or fifty drops of the tincture of opium, or one grain of

opium mixed with one and a half grains of ipecacuanha, to be repeated, if necessary, at the end of six hours. The powder is preferable to the tincture of opium in this case.

3. Sometimes the pains are not sufficiently strong to break the membranes containing the waters. If the presumption be, that the membranes are too rigid, or if sufficient time may have been allowed, it may become necessary to break them artificially. But as was observed under the head of Natural Labours, this must be done with the greatest caution. It should be first known, that the *os uteri* is fully dilated, and care must be taken, not to be deceived in this point, because the *os uteri* is sometimes so thinly and uniformly spread over the head of the child, before it is in any degree dilated, as very much to resemble the membranes.

If it be determined to break the membranes, no instrument is necessary but the finger, or at most the finger nail prepared for the purpose, by being cut and turned up.

4. The shortness of the funis or umbilical cord may be the cause of difficult labour, resembling that which is the effect of a feeble action of the womb, it may therefore be explained in this place. The umbilical cord may be short originally, or may be rendered so by being wound round the neck, body or

limbs of the child. If the child should be drawn back upon the declension of a pain, the shortness of the umbilical cord may be always suspected. By allowing sufficient time, this inconvenience will commonly be overcome. If however the child should not be born after waiting long enough, it may be necessary to change the position of the patient, and instead of reposing on a bed or couch, as advised in the instructions for *taking a pain*, she may be placed upon the lap of one of the assistants. *It will be frequently found advantageous to prefer this position in lingering cases, especially when the parts seem fully prepared for dilatation.*

When the head of the child is expelled, the funis may be brought forwards over the head, or backwards over the shoulders. But if neither can be done, it may be necessary to wait for the effects of more time. It is not so dangerous as some suppose, for the child to remain sometime in this position, but the air should have free access to its mouth. But when it can no longer be considered safe, the funis must be divided with the usual precaution of tying, &c.

5. If the child be dead and swelled, the labour will commonly be exceeding difficult, and put on appearances similar to those of the foregoing cases. It may be found neces-

sary in an instance of this sort, to pass a towel or handkerchief round the neck of the child, and then by taking hold of both ends, considerable aid may be afforded. But if this method should not succeed, one or both arms should be brought down and included in the handkerchief, by which means still greater force may be applied. In all cases however, where it can be done with safety, it will be more safe and humane to wait the effects of natural efforts, than to use much force.

6. Consumption and other diseases with general debility, commonly cause great apprehension about the issue of parturition. But if there is no untoward circumstance in the way, it will be found, that there is a peculiar balance obtaining between the strength of the patient, and the disposition of the parts concerned for dilatation; give them time and they will be delivered.

7. When labour is common, there is generally a sense of heat, quickness of the pulse, thirst, flushed cheeks, in one word a general feverish disposition. These appearances may be considered natural efforts, for carrying on the depending operations of the system. But the fever sometimes runs too high, and exhausts those powers of the system, which ought to have been otherwise applied. When

this is the case, nothing can be more erroneous, than the common and almost universal plan of giving wine, spirit, or other cordials. This kind of treatment is calculated to increase the fever, and destroy the pains. Instead of spirit, wine, or opium, have recourse to cooling drinks, and moderate blood letting; to be repeated according to circumstances. To these may be added frequent mild glysters, and a gentle purge or two. The room should be kept cool and well aired, and the patient as much as possible composed.

8. Fat and inactive women very frequently have slow and lingering labours, they seem subject to debility of the indirect kind. In every case of this sort it must be very improper to make use of spirits, &c. to hasten the pains.

9. Patients under the impression of fear, will in almost every instance be subject to a tedious labour, and as the time is prolonged, their fears will naturally increase, so that ultimately, they may be brought into danger by their own cowardly imagination. The midwife should therefore use discreet measures to inspire more favorable sentiments.

10. I will conclude this chapter with a general observation on the subject of letting blood in time of labour. It cannot be pro-

perly admissible in every case, even with the most robust women. But if there be fever, or if the pains be very strong, and the exertions of the woman seem vehement ; in either of these cases it is necessary to loose blood.

CHAPTER XIII.

SECOND KIND OF DIFFICULT LABOURS.

Most women with their first children, suffer more or less from the difficult distention of the parts concerned in parturition.. But the rigidity which is the cause, commonly lessens with every child, in proportion to the number which she has. Let sufficient time be allowed her, and the constitution will find sufficient resources within itself, for her delivery. Sometimes blood letting is necessary in this case.

If the woman be far advanced in age at the time of her having her first child, this rigidity of the parts will be the greater, and of course the labour may be the more difficult. Women of this description, might generally avoid much inconvenience, by occasional blood letting towards the close of pregnancy, by making frequent use of gentle laxatives, as manna, sweet oil, castor oil and the like, and by sitting over the steams of warm water, every night at bed time.* It may be observed however that it very frequently happens, that women at forty-five, fare as well as they could have done with a first child at twenty-five. None therefore ought to be discouraged. The natural efforts of the constitution in these cases are astonishing.

A difficulty of distention is frequently brought on by a premature rupture of the membranes containing the waters. When this circumstance takes place, whether the rupture be natural or artificial it sometimes happens, that many hours or even days may pass, before the accession of labour. In this case, it would be best for the patient, to continue most of her time lying in bed or on a couch.

The *os uteri* is sometimes removed from its central position. This may put on appearances similar to those of common rigidity. But no attempt should ever be made to change it by art. Nothing should be done, but direct the patient to lie much of her time on the side, towards which the *os uteri* is turned. Or if the *os uteri* be projected backwards, which is always the case,

---

* See the note at the close of the second part, page 73.

when it cannot be reached in the beginning or early part of labour, then the patient should lie much of her time upon her back.

The *os uteri* may be so rigid, as to require from twenty-four to forty hours for its dilatation, and yet no disorder be present. But it is sometimes made rigid by an inflammation of the part. This state of it may be known by its heat and dryness. And if the pains have long continued, without effect; and the principal difficulty be the resistance made by the *os uteri*, an inflammation may always be suspected.

To remove such inflammation let some blood be drawn, give every two hours forty drops of the spirits of nitre in a cup of some cooling tea, to which may be added one fifth of a grain of tartarized antimony, and mild glysters should be injected. Instead of giving any thing to raise the pains, keep the patient quiet in bed. Indeed a case might occur, in which the violence of the pains would force the *os uteri* down with the head of the child, unless she were carefully kept in a lying posture.

The rigidity of the external parts, is frequently the cause of difficult labour; but no artificial aid is allowed, but that advised under the head of natural labours.

CHAPTER XIV.

THIRD KIND OF DIFFICULT LABOURS.

If the pelvis be too small for the size of the child's head, it will obviously require the more time for bringing about the necessary changes for its passage. The same consequence will follow from a moderate degree of distortion, or narrowness of the pelvis. But as it is possible *for the head to be compressed into one third part of its dimensions*, it can of course pass through a passage, which would seem to be much too small. If however, the distortion be very great, or the head be of such a degree of strength, as to prevent a passage entirely; then the women must be delivered by the aid of instruments; otherwise she must perish together with the child. But instruments ought to be introduced with caution, and in no case before time, with other circumstances prove them to be necessary. And then a surgeon should be employed.

If the head of the child should be uncommonly large, similar difficulties will follow. But this may be also overcome by the natural efforts, if sufficient time be allowed. In some cases the head is so enlarged by disease, that it may be necessary to open it with an instrument. But as the head when distended with water, sometimes bursts from the pressure of the pains, this operation ought not to be too hastily performed.

If the face of the child be turned towards the *pubis*, the labour will commonly be tedious. But generally no artificial aid is wanting; more time must be allowed for the descent of the child, and more care will be required, when it passes through the external parts. The case would be similar, if the face should present.

A difficult labour, similar to that in consequence of a narrow pelvis, will take place when one or both arms present together with the head. Where it can be done, the arms should be put back and carefully detained. "In some cases of this kind, the head, an arm, and a foot may be all felt at the same time. When this happens, it is best to grasp and bring down the foot, and deliver in that manner."

When a child is born, with one or both arms presenting together with the head, the arm or arms will be much bruised, and will demand attention. They should be bathed in vinegar and water, or spirit and water, and soft poultices of some kind should be applied.

CHAPTER XV.

FOURTH KIND OF DIFFICULT LABOURS.

Every precaution ought to be taken to prevent too great a distention of the bladder; for if the urine should collect in large quantities, it will not only be a hindrance to the labour, but the pain may become so great as to do much injury. If all precaution fail, a catheter must be used to draw off the water where it can be done.

Should there be a large stone in the bladder, or an adhesion of the vagina, so as to prevent the passage of the child, a surgeon ought to be immediately called in.

If a large unnatural substance should grow out of the *os uteri*, and obstruct the passage, it may be necessary to lessen the head of the child, by letting out its contents.

Scars in the vagina from past injury, will generally yield to the natural efforts of the constitution.

Sometimes the womb itself is ruptured. If this truly alarming circumstance should take place, it may be readily known. The patient will perceive distinctly a sense of something giving way internally, with a sudden excruciating pain in some part of the abdomen. An instant vomiting of whatever the stomach may contain will follow, which will commonly be a fluid of a brown colour. An abatement or total cessation of *the pains* will take place, and there will be a discharge of blood from the vagina. In addition to these symptoms, the limbs of the child may be felt, by applying the hand to the abdomen. The patient commonly dies though not always immediately. A case has occurred, where the child was turned after the rupture of the womb, and safely delivered to the preservation of both mother and child. This ought therefore always to be tried.

The cases of difficult labour admit of great variety, and much practice is necessary for preparing any one to treat every case to the best advantage. Regard should be had to the cause of the difficulty, which should be ascertained if possible, because a knowledge of this would afford aid in determining the proper mode of procedure. Here I must be permitted to repeat my assertion, that the greater number of difficult labours, are not such from unavoidable necessity, but are rendered difficult, from some improper management in the beginning, or through the course of labour. The midwife may sometimes err, the patient may be intractable, and the impatience, and unseasonable anxiety of her friends, may lead them to demand improper treatment.

CHAPTER XVI.

INSTRUMENTS, &c.

Several instruments have been invented for aiding in difficult labours, as the *forceps*, *vectis*, *fillet*, *&c.* but as they ought not be used except in cases of great necessity, and then by those only, who are well acquainted with instrumental delivery; I shall not attempt at a description of them. Such midwives however, as are desirous of being acquainted with this part of the art, are referred to the late work of Dr. Thomas Denman, where they may find a very distinct and intelligent account of their figure, and the manner of applying them in practice, &c. From this excellent treatise, a very great proportion of these hints are extracted, some in the language of Dr. Denman; others with considerable variation, as I found it most convenient to my design.

CHAPTER XVII.

PRETERNATURAL LABOURS.

Preternatural labours may be divided into two orders.

I. When the breech or lower extremities present.

II. When the shoulders or upper extremities present.

Natural and difficult labours are considered, as having reference chiefly to the mother.

But preternatural labours are considered, as having reference to the position of the child.

It therefore is obvious, that a preternatural labour may happen to a woman in perfect health, who has every possible regularity in her formation, and who may have passed through all the common changes of parturition, in the most favourable manner.

Different opinions have been entertained concerning the causes of preternatural presentation, but none of them is sufficiently clear and certain, to be of any advantage in directing the conduct by which they may be prevented.

Various symptoms too have been as stated as indicating such a presentation. But it cannot be certainly known, until the part presenting can be felt and distinguished by the touch. The *head* may be known by its roundness and firmness. The *breech* by the cleft between the buttocks and by the parts of generation. A *hand* by the thumb and length of the fingers. And a *foot* by the heel and its want of a thumb.

CHAPTER XVIII.

FIRST ORDER OF PRETERNATURAL LABOURS.

In the first order of preternatural labours may be included, the presentation of the breech; of a hip; of the knees; and of one or both legs.

When a labour is so far advanced, that the *os uteri* is fully dilated, if no part of the child can be felt, it will be prudent to watch carefully for the rupture of the membranes; because it may be that the child ought to be immediately turned; and if it be done quickly after the waters are evacuated it may be effected with ease, but if delayed a very little time, the uterus will contract, after which it is done with considerable difficulty. So soon as the membranes are broken, it will be proper to introduce the hand, and make the necessary examination. Should the head or breech present, the hand may be withdrawn, and the labour suffered to proceed without interruption, as a natural presentation. But when the breech presents, great attention is required in conducting the body in such a manner, as to secure a safe passage for the head. For if the face be towards the pubis, it must be managed so as gradually to turn it, till one ear shall be towards the pubis, the other towards the sacrem.

If it be found, that the child will pass readily enough with its arms turned up, there will be no occasion to bring them down, but if the head remain fixed, after using the force which is thought safe and prudent to be exerted, the arms should be brought down. Care should be used, not to break or dislocate the bones of the child, or injure the external parts of the mother.

If there be difficulty after the arms are brought down, the finger might be passed into the mouth of the child, and its lower jaw be turned upon its breast, taking care not to pull by it. By this change of the position of the head, the passage may be more readily effected. Should necessity require it, the body of the child may be moved in different directions; that is from side to side, up and down, using it as a lever for the extraction of the head; but it must be done with all care and tenderness.

But it may happen that after giving full scope and due time, to the natural efforts of the mother, they prove ineffectual for the expulsion of the child. Assistance must be then given her. As the breech is supposed to present, a finger may be locked in the groin, and such force used as may be deemed sufficient to extract it without injury. If this should not do, a ribband or piece of tape may be passed over one or both thighs, with which considerable force may be used with greater safety to the mother and child.

In all cases of this kind it is necessary to have particular regard to the umbilical cord. It should never be on the stretch or it will be highly injurious to the child.

CHAPTER XIX.

SECOND ORDER OF PRETERNATURAL LABOURS.

If the shoulder, or one or both arms present, there is a necessity of turning the child and delivering by the feet. This second order of preternatural labours, admits of four variations.

1. The first is, where the os uteri being fully dilated, and the membranes unbroken, a superior extremity is felt through them: Or where such preternatural presentation is discovered immediately upon the rupture of the membranes and the discharge of the waters, before there is any return of the pains,

or any contraction of the uterus round the body of the child. In this case the mangem nt is simple and easy. The patient is to be placed in the same situation as in a natural labour ; upon her left side, with her knees drawn up across the bed, and as near to the edge of it as possible. Every practitioner however ought to choose that position, in which he or she can probably perform with the greatest dexterity. The patient being placed, if the external parts be not sufficiently dilated, the fingers of the right hand must be reduced into the form of a sugar loaf, by placing them together around the thumb, and with the hand in this form, the dilation must be sufficiently effected. But this operation should be performed very slowly, so as to resemble the natural dilation as much as possible. When the hand can readily pass thro' the external parts, it must be conducted slowly to the os uteri. If the membranes be not broken, they must be grasped firmly so as to rupture them ; or they may be perforated with the finger. Then let the hand be carried cautiously along the sides, thighs and legs of the child, till it comes to the feet, and if possible, by a firm grasp and waving motion, let both feet be brought down together. Waiting then for a return of the pains, they may be brought a little lower, and so on, till they pass the external parts. By observing the toes it may be told whether the back of the child be towards the pubis, which is the proper position. The assistance to be afterwards afforded may be regulated accordingly. The feet may be wrapped in a cloth, so as to be held firmly and used as may be afterwards found most convenient; as in chap. XVIII. Section third.

2. The second variation of this order, may include those cases, in which at the time of the rupture of the membranes, there is very little dilatation of the os uteri, and some degree of contraction of the os uterus.

As there is danger of doing mischief by every artificial dilatation of the os uteri, it will be best to wait, till it dilates in the natural way. It may not be necessary to wait however till the dilatation is quite complete, but only till it will admit the hand readily. Then with some additional difficulty, it may be conducted as before. In the mean time if the dilatation is delayed from an inflammatory affection of the parts, the treatment must be similar to that advised in chap. XIII. section 5.

3. The third variation may include those cases in which, together with the presentation of an arm or shoulder, there is the worst possible situation of the child in all other re-

spects; as a close contraction of the uterus round the body of the child; the membranes having been long broken and the waters discharged; and in addition to the whole, very strong pains. In treating this case I will be particular. It is improper to be in a hurry, as though whatever could be done must be executed in haste. Such conduct would greatly alarm the patient, and make the matter worse. Let a very accurate examination be made, in the most deliberate manner. A correct judgment should be formed of the presentation. It should also be determined to which side the feet lie, and this last may be known by the situation of the palm of the hand, which always naturally turns towards the feet.

Having made the necessary examination, the contraction of the womb must next be moderated. And this must be done, whether the contraction be continued, or alternate as in natural pains, or irregular resembling cramp. For this purpose, if she be much heated, let blood be drawn and the bleeding repeated according to circumstances. Give one, two, or more mild glysters, and use such language and conduct as may tend to soothe the patient. When she seems to be in some degree composed, give her two or three grains of opium. In the course of twenty or thirty minutes, she will be easy or sleepy, and then will be the time to proceed to the operation of turning.

It should always be remembered, that so much force must be used, as may be necessary to overcome the contraction of the womb, which constantly prevails. But when there is alternate contraction and partial relaxation, the hand must stop during the contraction, and it must be spread out smoothly to prevent a rupture of the womb. In other respects proceed as in the second variation of this order.

Sometimes the shoulder of the child is so jammed at the upper part of the pelvis, that the hand is prevented from passing. In that case, the fore finger and thumb must be used in the form of a crutch under the armpit of the child, to push the shoulder towards the head and towards the upper part of the uterus. However great the difficulty, composure and perseverance are necessary. If the first, or any number of efforts fail, they still may be preparing the way for future success. Sometimes in consequence of the particular kind of contraction of the uterus, it may be so lengthened out, as to make it difficult to reach the feet. In such a case on finding the knees, the legs and feet may be brought down together; and here again care must be taken, that an arm be not mistaken for a foot. The feet when found may be brought down slowly, and for the greater safety a ribbon may be fixed over the wrist in a noose, before the hand is introduced, and when the feet are brought low enough, the noose may be slipped with the fingers of the left hand over the feet, which will thus be secured. If the body of the child be fixed across the upper part of the pelvis, great aid will be found to arise from holding the two ends of the noose in the right hand, while with the finger and thumb of the left, in the form of a crutch in the armpit of the child, its body may be raised till it is disengaged, and there is room for the entrance of the hips into the pelvis. The remainder of the operation as before.

4. The fourth variation implies the foregoing difficulties, but in addition may take in the case of a distortion of the pelvis; and here the greatest difficulty attends the extraction of the head. Having therefore proceeded through the whole operation as described in the other variations, at length the whole of the child is born except the head. While in this situation, the child is in great danger from the compression of the *funis*. But if there be a vigorous pulsation in the funis there is no danger, and hurry will be improp-

er. Should the pulsation however which was at first lively and strong, gradually decline, and then altogether cease, the head must be immediately extracted, or the child will inevitably be lost. If there be reason to expect the preservation of the child, the force applied must be moderate and cautious, it must be exerted in a proper direction with regard to the pelvis, it must be uniform and commanded, and if there be any pains, it must accompany them. If there be no prospect of saving the child still more time may be employed. After using as much force as may be consistent with the mother's safety, it will be proper to rest awhile, that the head may be compressed and adapted to the pelvis. And thus, by acting and resting alternately, with efficacy and resolution, the delivery may at length be completed. But if the hold which may be had of the body do not suit, a silk handkerchief or ribbon may be passed round its neck, and by this aid the necessary force may readily be applied.— By pursuing this plan with firmness, resting at proper intervals, it must indeed be a very difficult case if it be not at length overcome.

In all cases where the head is extracted with difficulty, it should be remembered that by too violent force the head may be separated from the body. With proper moderation and care this accident will seldom happen.—When it does occur, the head must be lessened. This may be safely and readily enough performed, if an assistant confine the head against the upper part of the pelvis, by applying the hand upon the abdomen, with a firm and equal pressure till the opening is made, and till some proper instrument be fastened upon it ; this being done, with the usual precautions the head may be safely extracted.

CHAPTER XX.

COMPLEX LABOURS.

Complex labours admit of four orders.

I. Labours attended with flooding.

II. Labours attended with convulsions.

III. Labours with two or more children.

IV. Labours where the umbilical cord descends before any part of the child.

The first order admits four variations.

1. Those which happen in early pregnancy, commonly called abortions.

2. Those which occur in advanced pregnancy, or at the full periods of gestation.

3. Those which happen between the birth of the child, and the expulsion of the placenta.

4. Those which follow the expulsion of the placenta.

CHAPTER XXI.

I. FLOODINGS IN ABORTION.

If the fœtus be expelled at any time before the end of the sixth month, it may be called an abortion. But an expulsion in any of the last three months, may be considered a labour premature or irregular.

Cases of abortion neither require nor admit of any manual assistance ; for the proper treatment in this case see chap. XXIV. part II.

But when a woman is miscarrying with a considerable and apparently dangerous flooding, is so far advanced in pregnancy that it may be difficult to determine, whether the case be an abortion or a premature labour ; the circumstances being such at the same time as to render it unsafe to depend on the common remedies, it may become necessary to hasten her delivery. For this purpose the membranes may be broken and the waters discharged. By this evacuation, the uterus will be made to contract, and the flooding will be stayed until the *foetus* can be expelled by the natural efforts of the constitution.

It is worthy of observation, that in some instances, the fœ us at an earlier stage of pregnancy, is found hanging in the os uteri, where it might remain if neglected, and continue to be the cause of a long and dangerous flooding. In lingering cases, this ought at least to be suspected, and if discovered, the foetus should be moved a little in different directions, so as to hasten its expulsion : Remembering at the same time, that it must be done in the gentlest manner possible.

CHAPTER XXII.

PREMATURE LABOURS WITH FLOODING.

In premature labours great and dangerous floodings may be induced, either by the placenta being attached over the *os uteri*, or by a separation of a part or the whole of the placenta, so as to leave the open blood vessels in a state of distention.

The first may be discovered by a fleshy substance without any part of the membranes, which presents on a common examination : And the second may be known, by being able to distinguish the membranes without any such fleshy substance. Although there is danger in either case, yet the first is most to be dreaded. The danger however is to be determined, not by the supposed quantity of blood lost, but by the effect produced on the patient, one person can loose much more than another.

Danger is indicated by weakness and quickness of the pulse, or by the pulse becoming and continuing imperceptible; by coldness and paleness of the body, and by a ghastly countenance; by restlessness and continual faintings; by short and difficult breathing, and by convulsions. Sometimes the patient is taken with a sudden and violent fit of vomiting, this is commonly beneficial. Floodings with pain, are less dangerous than those in which the patient seems to be at ease.

Having therefore used every precaution, and observed carefully the state of the patient, so as neither to be too hasty nor too late in affording assistance, and with the greatest deliberation having determined that she ought to be delivered by art, in order to preserve her life, let her be placed as before directed, then let the parts be dilated with great caution, so as readily to admit the hand. If the placenta be attached over the *os uteri* it is of no consequence whether it be separated, so as to come to its edge and go up on the outside of the membranes, which may be ruptured at pleasure ; or whether a perforation be made through the substance of the placenta. In either case, with regard to the position of the child, its feet should be found, and with a slow waving motion brought down as advised in chap. XIX.

If the placenta be not attached over the *os uteri*, but the flooding is the consequence of a partial separation, and the case be urgent, let the membranes be ruptured, observing the kind of presentation ; and where circumstances seem favourable, the remaining part of the operation may be left to the constitution. But if the symptoms be urgent and the danger great every part of the proceeding must be the more expeditious.

CHAPTER XXIII.

FLOODING AFTER THE BIRTH BEFORE THE EXPULSION OF THE PLACENTA.

Whenever it can be safely done, the placenta ought to be excluded in the natural way, see part III. chap. X. But if there be dangerous flooding, it must be immediately extracted.* Pressure on the abdomen, gen-

* It is too commonly the case that the friends of the patient together with the midwife, elated with joy at

the pulling of the funis, a change of her position, &c. &c. are first to be employed, but if these fail, the hand must be introduced. If however the flooding should have already proceeded so far as to induce fainting and the like, the patient must be somewhat revived before the operation.

Whenever it is determined to proceed, the patient being placed in a convenient position, the funis is to be held in the one hand, with a moderate degree of tightness, while the other is to be guided by the funis through the vagina, os uteri, &c. into the uterus. Whatever dilatation is to be artificially made, must be effected carefully ; and when the placenta is examined, so as to determine its degree of attachment, the procedure must be regulated accordingly. Sometimes the irritation excited by the introduction of the hand, brings about the separation without any farther aid. But if the attachment be complete, grasp the placenta between all the fingers. If no part is separated by this attempt, the edge must be found and carefully raised. Then with the blunt end of the fingers, continue the sep-

---

the happy deliverance of the child, demand an immediate extraction of the cake. Hundreds have been destroyed by this barbarous custom. The natural efforts ought always to be permitted to expel this also as well as the child.

aration in a slow and cautious manner. When the separation is thought to be sufficiently effected for the purpose, grasp it again and gently bear it off towards the adhering edge till it is quite separated. Then wait till the womb begins to contract, which may be roused into action, if seemingly inactive, by throwing the fingers back gently against its side. Then bring the placenta down into the vagina, where let it stay at least one hour, unless sooner expelled by the natural efforts of the system. These directions with some variations, can be adapted to almost any case that may occur.

CHAPTER XXIV.

FLOODING AFTER THE EXPULSION OF THE PLACENTA.

The cautions advised above, will generally prevent any dangerous loss of blood. But if by any means the uterus has been inverted, it will probably be the cause of an alarming and long continued flooding. By external examination with the hand applied on the abdomen, and by actual examination by the vagina, it ought to be ascertained whether the womb be inverted, and if it be, it should be speedily, but cautiously replaced, afterwards the usual remedies would be successful, but never before. If the uterus should be inverted while the placenta or a part of it adheres, this should first be separated, and then the uterus may be carefully and gently replaced.

CHAPTER XXV.

II. *LABOURS WITH CONVULSION.*

Where the patient is afflicted with slight delirium, swimming and violent pain of the head, blindness, pain or cramp at the stomach, chills with every return of the pains, great and excessive vomitings, &c. there is danger of convulsions.

Convulsions which attend parturition differ in some respects from all others. The most obvious symptoms of this kind of convulsions, are a contraction of the muscles, distortion of the eyes, twitchings, foaming of the mouth, &c. as in epilepsy, but there will also be a snoring like that attendant on apoplexy, and she will make a hissing noise as if she were drawing her spittle through her teeth. By observing the cautions and advice given in part II. convulsions may generally be prevented. But if they should take place the patient should be bled largely, if possible from the jugular or neck veins, if this cannot be done, blood letting from the arm must be repeated as often as may be necessary. From two to five pints may be drawn in the course of a few hours, and when properly and sufficiently employed, blood letting seldom fails.

After bleeding, the warm bath, or where that cannot be employed, clothes wrung out of warm water may be applied all over the abdomen with similar effects. But it may be remembered that the patient ought not to be delivered by art, in consequence of the convulsions, without first having regard to all the precautions given in the cases heretofore explained.

CHAPTER XXVI.

III. LABOURS WITH TWO OR MORE CHILDREN.

There are no certain marks by which it can be foretold that a woman carries twins. Neither an unusual size, nor uncommon sensation about the uterus, nor any particular discharge of the waters, nor the slowness of the progress of labour, affords any information worth attention. But after the birth of the first child, it may be determined by applying the hand to the abdomen. It must be a very good rule to keep patients who have borne one child ignorant of there being another as long as it can be done. But in most instances after the birth of the first child, the second will follow in a few minutes with great rapidity. The whole progress will generally be the same as if there were but the one child. But if the first one must be turned, it will require care not to break the membranes of the second, if they be yet whole. If the first be excluded safely, there cannot often be any difficulty in the exclusion of the second. If the first be delivered by art, the presumption is, the second will require similar management. Should the pains be suspended after the birth of the first, the second should be suffered to remain at least four hours before artificial aid be introduced. But if convulsions or floodings take place, no more time must be delayed, than the state of the case would warrant.

In twin cases, the two cakes are usually united, so as to form one mass, though they are sometimes distinct. But whether separate or united, no attempt should be made to extract the placenta of the first till both children are born. When the second child is extracted by art, it is frequently the case, that the placenta must also be extracted by art, and if one must be so extracted the other ought not to be left behind, because a flooding might be the consequence.

CHAPTER XXVII.

IV. LABOURS WHERE THERE IS A DESCENT OF THE UMBILICAL CORD BEFORE THE CHILD.

If the umbilical cord should happen to descend before any part of the child, it cannot endanger the mother, but it necessarily places the child in jeopardy. If it can be returned and kept back, it ought to be done. If this cannot be effected, it should be placed to one side, so as to avoid compression. For on a continuance of its circulation depends the life of the child. Or if it be deemed more safe and prudent, the os uteri being fully dilated, the child may be turned. But by the state of the umbilical cord it must first be determined, whether the child be living or dead; for if it be dead, the labour ought to be suffered to proceed. So also if the funis descend before the os uteri is dilated, the presumption is that whatever aid could be afforded would be fruitless, therefore the labour ought not to be interrupted.

CHAPTER XXVIII.

MANAGEMENT OF WOMEN IN CHILDBED.

After delivery give the patient suitable refreshment and leave her to repose. There should be as little change as possible from her former habits and customs, either in diet or in any other respect. Let her drink be cool, and her food adapted to the state of her case. If she be very faint, a little wine might be allowed, but in common cases spirits of every kind are pernicious.

Pains sometimes occur for the purpose of excluding the clotted blood, which may be lodged in the uterus. These are salutary of course, and ought not to be entirely stopped, if it could be done. But they will be more effectual and moderate, if one or more stools be procured pretty soon after delivery, by injecting a glyster or two. Also a cloth wrung out of warm water, may be applied to the abdomen. After the proper evacuations, if the warm cloth does not afford relief, small doses of opium may be given.

For a soreness of the abdomen, a warm flannel sprinkled with spirits of some kind may be applied. It should be large enough to cover the affected parts, and should be occasionally removed. Pain in the bowels should be removed by a gentle purge. And in those cases, where the labour has been difficult and the patient tolerably robust, as also in cases of a common kind when the lochial discharge is in any degree deficient, it would be prudent to give a pretty brisk purge, varied according to the strength of the patient. Jalap and calomel might be used to advantage with this intention.

Strict regard should be had to cleanliness, both as it regards the person and cloathing of the patient. And her mind should be kept as cheerful as possible. Without these precautions, and sometimes notwithstanding all possible care, the following dangerous fever may take place.

CHAPTER XXIX.

PUERPERAL, OR CHILD-BED FEVER.

The puerperal fever comes on gradually, beginning from twenty hours to thirty days, and sometimes as many weeks after delivery. Weak and delicate women, and especially those accustomed to genteel life, are most subject to it. It begins with a chill, and the symptoms attending it, are, nausea, pain in the head, loss of strength, and restlessness.

The skin is sometimes dry, at other times partially or unusually moist. The tongue is dry, and sometimes covered with a black crust. The pulse varies being sometimes weak and small, and then again full and tense. Wandering pains are felt in the abdomen, and sometimes they attack the sides, resembling pleurisy. In some cases they extend to the shoulder blade, to the short ribs, liver and spleen, then descend to the bladder and lower intestines. The pain becomes so acute in some instances, that the patient cannot bear the weight of the bed clothes. The face has a sorrowful appearance, and every word and action will more or less express her sufferings both of body and mind. Sometimes the belly swells as in pregnancy. Pains are felt in the back and buttocks, the legs swell, and at length the breathing becomes difficult. So great will be the loss of strength that she will be unable to turn in bed. Vomiting and diarrhea, and sometimes a stubborn costivenens takes place. The lochia are sometimes suppressed, at other times they continue throughout the disease, and when the inflammation is confined to the uterus this must be a favourable circumstance. The urine is scanty, is frequently evacuated, and is turbid. Spots appear on the joints. It continues from three to five days, and sometimes in the country to ten, fifteen and twenty days. Although the appearances vary in different patients, yet by this catalogue of symptoms, the puerperal fever may be known. And if it should occur, a physician should be immediately called in. But if none can be obtained, on the first attack the patient should be bled, according to her strength and the violence of the attack. Then a mild vomit of fifteen grains of ipecacuanha, with one quarter or one half grain of tartarized antimony should be given. And after a gentle evacuation downwards an opiate at night.— Glysters, fomentations, and an opening draught of senna, manna and cream of tartar combined, may be daily repeated. If the disease be prolonged for several days, it is the more necessary that a physician should be called in, because bleeding in the common way might do harm. But where the propriety of bleeding is doubtful, an emetic might generally be given with safety. If there be frequent or involuntary stools caution is necessary not to administer any thing which may do injury. In such case, glysters of chicken water, or flour and water boiled to a proper consistence, or flaxseed tea ought to be often repeated. It requires judgment to determine the propriety of correcting this diarrhea. If however it becomes necessary through the debility of the patient to check it, an infusion of columbo root, or flowers of camomile may be used, as also the starch glyster with the addition of fifty drops of the tincture of opium. Should a hiccuping come on, take spirits of nitre one quarter of an ounce, clean water one half pint, and white sugar at discretion. Of this mixture give two spoonfuls every two or three hours.—She should breathe pure air. Strict regard should be had to cleanliness. Her rest must be secured, and silence should be carefully preserved. It is thought, not without good reason, that this fever may be communicated by contagion. This circumstance will make it necessary for the midwife to be cautious in every respect, so as not to convey it from one to another.

CHAPTER XXX.

DISEASES OF LESS IMPORTANCE.

1. Swelled legs. A very distressing and painful swelling of the legs sometimes follows parturition. In some cases it affects one leg only, and in others it seizes upon both. Apply to the swelled limb night and morning an ointment made of an ounce of

olive oil, and an ounce of camphor. If there be debility an infusion of columbo or camomile might be used till the strength of the patient be recovered. If there be fever treat it as at chap. XXIX.

2. SWELLED BREARTS. Are relieved by an ointment of olive oil and camphor as above, or the ley poultice of a moderate strength, or mercurial ointment, and finally the lancet.

3. SORE NIPPLES. Are to be relieved by an application of Turlington's balsam, balsam peru, lead water, or by drawing the breast three or four weeks before and after delivery. If blood should be discharged from the breast instead of milk, give the jesuits bark and wash the breast with port wine.

Sometimes a solution of borax is very beneficial as an application to sore nipples. It ought to be tried.

END OF THE THIRD PART.

Part Fourth.

An essay on the management and common diseases of children.

CHAPTER I.

INTRODUCTION.

IN the first part of this work, a heavy task is imposed on the mother; so heavy indeed that I could not have expected her performance of it, if my eye had not been turned upon the great and continual aid, which she ought to receive from her husband. Let no man think to excuse himself from this interesting duty. Whatever may be his occupation; however important his calling in life, he is bound by self love, by parental affection, and by that patriotic interest which every good man feels in the rising generation, to devote a considerable part of his attention to the government, and instruction of his children.

" He is bound by self love," It is an excellent institution, that children bear their father's name. Not only as it assists in the distribution and descent of property, but as it becomes a powerful motive in favor of education. If posterity be infamous, they brand disgrace on the name they bear; if respectable, they reflect honor upon their respective families.

"He is bound by parental affection." The great tenderness felt by both parents for their infant offspring is no doubt intended to urge them to take measures for the welfare of the darling babe. Experience might teach us, that a man of correct taste, could not maintain a warm regard for a perverse and disagreeable child. To love a son or daughter merely as being ours, though destitute of all merit, must surely require very strong animal attachment. But the proper steps being taken to form him worthy of esteem, parents find themselves daily rewarded in their success. As the child becomes more amiable, their attachment which at first is altogether instinctive and considerably selfish, gradually changes its form from the animal to the rational kind. Hence they are at length prepared to practice self denial and encounter every difficulty to secure to their child a tranquil life.

"He is bound by the interest he feels in the rising generation." If a man deserves the honorable appellation of *a lover of his country*, his patriotism will first appear in his attachment to his family, and in the attention he pays to the education of his children. Let him make the greatest pretensions to public spirit! and utter the loudest declamations for the public good! If he be deficient in his parental duties, his *love of country* is mere ostentation. He is at best *an office hunter*.

The prosperity of a nation may be determined by its population, which, if it be the greatest possible, necessarily implies the highest degree of civilization. Hence the manners of a nation have a powerful influence on its prosperity. The national character must ultimately be resolved into that of families and individuals. Every true patriot must therefore feel himself bound to add to the public stock of respectability and happiness, as well his own best example, as the additional number of good citizens to be raised up under his government and protection, in the capacity of the *father of a family*.

There is another consideration of still greater importance with those who have faith in divine revelation. Believing all men to be accountable to the GREAT GOD who will judge the world in righteousness. Contemplating every soul of man born into the world, as a candidate for immortal bliss or endless woe. Knowing that present and future happiness depends on the formation of those tempers of mind which were in CHRIST JESUS. The christain will feel himself compelled by the fear of God, by the love of truth, and by the consolations of the gospel, to be instant in his exertions to prepare his children through divine assistance for the kingdom of heaven.

CHAPTER II.

AGREEMENT OF PARENT'S NECESSARY.

Doctor Witherspoon in his letters on education says " Husband and wife ought to be entirely one upon this subject; not only agreed as to the end, but as to the means to be used, and the plan to be followed, in order to attain it. If their opinions happen to differ in any particular, they ought to examine the matter privately by themselves and settle it, so that not the least opposition may appear to the children or servants." Such unanimity will be of great importance in the government of a family. " It will enforce every rule by a double authority, and recommend it by a double example." Without this consent, their labours must be more than lost, not only failing to do good, but necessarily producing much evil.

"These observations are by no means intended against those unhappy couples, who being essentially different in principles and character, live in a state of continual war. It is of little advantage to speak either to or of such persons; but even differences incomparable smaller, are of very bad consequence. When one for example thinks a child may be carried out, and the other thinks it is wrong; when one thinks a way of speaking is dangerous, and the other is positive there is nothing in it; the things themselves may be of little moment, but the want of concurrence in the parents, or the want of mutual esteem and deference easily observed even by very young children, is of the greatest importance."

CHAPTER III

ABSOLUTE AUTHORITY OF PARENTS OVER THEIR CHILDREN NECESSARY.

In Part I. chap. II. I have laid it down as a fundamental proposition, "that the reason and experience of parents should be employed in the government of their children through the whole course of their infancy." Most children manifest a disposition to exert their will in opposition to that of their parents before they are twelve months old; and the more they are indulged, the more perverse they grow, till at length their insolence and petulence become intolerable. As soon as possible therefore an entire and absolute authority should be established over them. "I would have it early, says the doctor, that it may be absolute, and absolute that it may not be severe. If parents should be too long in beginning to exert their authority, they will find the task very difficult. Children habituated to indulgence for a few of their first years, are exceedingly impatient of restraint, and if they happen to be of stiff or obstinate tempers, can hardly be brought to an entire, at least to a quiet and placid submission. Whereas if they are taken in time, there is hardly any temper but what may be made to yield, and by early habit the subjection becomes quite easy to themselves.

The authority ought also to be absolute, that it may not be severe. "The more complete and uniform a parent's authority is, the offences will be more rare; punishment will be less needed, and the more gentle kind of correction will be abundantly sufficient; we see every where about us examples of this. A parent that has once obtained, and knows how to preserve authority, will do more by a look of displeasure, than another by the most passionate words and even blows. It holds universally in families and schools, and even in the greatest bodies of men, the army and navy, that those who keep the strictest discipline, give the fewest strokes. I have frequently remarked, that parents, even of the softest tempers, and who are famed for the greatest indulgence to their children, do, notwithstanding correct them more frequently, and even more severely, though to very little purpose, than those who keep up their authority. The reason is plain. Children by foolish indulgence, become often so froward and petulent in their tempers, that they provoke their easy parents past all endurance; so that they are obliged, if not to strike, at least to scold them, in a manner as little to their own credit, as children's profit."

"There is not a more disgusting sight than the impotent rage of a parent who has no authority. Among the lower ranks of people, who are under no restraint from decency, you may sometimes see a father or mother running out into the street after a child who is fled from them, with looks of fury and words of execration, and they are often stupid enough to imagine that neighbours or passengers will approve them in their conduct, though in fact it fills every beholder with horror. There is a degree of the same fault to be seen in persons of better rank, though expressing itself somewhat differently. Ill words and altercations will often fall out between parents and children before company, a sure sign that there is a defect of government at home, or in private. The parent stung with shame at the misbehaviour or indiscretion of the child, desires to persuade the observers that it is not his fault, and thereby convinces every person of reflection that it is."

CHAPTER IV.

THE BEST AND MILDEST WAY TO ESTABLISH THE NECESSARY AUTHORITY.

"I would recommend to every parent to begin the establishment of authority much more early than is commonly supposed to be possible: that is to say, from about the age of eight or nine months; you will perhaps smile at this, but I do assure you from experience, that by setting about it with prudence, deliberation, and attention, it may be in a manner completed by the age of twelve or fourteen months. Do not imagine that I mean to bid you use the rod at that age; on the contrary, I mean to prevent the use of it in a great measure, and to point out a way by which children of sweet and easy tempers may be brought to such a habit of compliance, as never to need correction at all; and whatever their tempers may be, so much less of this is sufficient, than upon any other supposition. This is one of my favorite schemes, let me try to explain and recommend it."

"Habits in general may be very early formed in children; an association of ideas is, as it were the parent of habit. If then you can accustom your children to perceive that your *will* must always prevail over theirs when they are opposed, the thing is done, and they will submit to it without difficulty or regret."

"To bring this about, as soon as they begin to show their inclination by desire or aversion, let single instances be chosen now and then (not too frequently) to contradict them. For example, if a child show a desire to have any thing in his hand with which he is delighted, let the parent take it from him and when he does so, let no consideration whatever make him restore it at that time. Then at a considerable interval, perhaps a whole day is little enough, especially at first, let the same thing be repeated. In the mean time it must be carefully observed, that no attempt should be made to contradict the child in the intervals. Not the least appearance of opposition, if possible, should be found between the will of the parent and that of the child, except in those chosen cases, when the parent must always prevail.

"I think it necessary that those attempts should always be made and repeated at proper intervals by the same person. It is also better it should be by the father, than the mother or any female attendant, because they will necessarily be obliged in many cases to do things displeasing to the child, as in dressing, washing, &c. which spoil the operation. Neither is it necessary that they should interpose, for when once a full authority is established in one person it can easily be communicated to others, as far as it is proper. Remember, however, that mother or nurse should never presume to condole with the child, or shew any signs of displeasure at his being crossed; but on the contrary, give every mark of approbation, and of their own submission to the same person.

"This experiment frequently repeated, will in a little time so perfectly habituate the child to yield to the parent, whenever he interposes, that he will make no opposition. I can assure you from experience, having literally practiced this method myself, that I never had a child of twelve months old but who would suffer me to take any thing from him or her, without the least mark of anger or dissatisfaction; while they would not suffer any other to do so, without the bitterest complaints. You will easily perceive how this is to be extended gradually, from one thing to another, from contradicting to commanding, &c."

This theory of Dr. Witherspoon is pleasing and interesting. It is also practical as I well know from my own experience. But its importance in establishing an early and absolute authority over children, will further appear from the following considerations, taken from the same excellent letters.

"There is a great diversity in the temper and disposition of children; and no less in the penetration, precedence and resolution of parents. From these circumstances, difficulties arise, which encrease very fast as the work is delayed. Some children have naturally very stiff and obstinate tempers, and some have a certain pride, or if you please, greatness of mind, which makes them think it a mean thing to yield. This disposition is often greatly strengthened in those of high birth, by the ideas of their own dignity and importance instilled into them from their mothers milk. I have known a boy of six years of age, who made it a point of honor not to cry when he was beat even by his parents. Other children have so strong passions, or so great sensibility, that if they receive correction, they will cry immoderately, and either be, or seem to be affected to such a degree, as to endanger their health or life. Neither is it uncommon for the parents in such a case to give up the point, and if they do not ask pardon, they give very genuine marks of repentance and sorrow for what they have done. I have said this is not uncommon, but I may rather ask, whether you know any parents at all, who have so much prudence and firmness, as not to be discouraged in the one case or to relent in the other? But it must always be remembered that the correction is wholly lost which does not produce absolute submission. Perhaps I may say that it is more than lost, because it will irritate instead of reforming them, and will instruct or perfect them in the art of overcoming their parents, which they will not fail to manifest on a future opportunity. It is surprising to think, how early children will discover the weak side of their parents, and what ingenuity they will shew in obtaining their favor or avoiding their displeasure. I think I have observed a child in treaty or expostulation with a parent, discover more consummate policy at seven years of age, than the parent himself, even when attempting to cajole him with artful evasions and specious promises. On all these accounts, it must be a vast advantage, that a habit of submission should be brought on so early, that even memory itself shall not be able to reach back to its beginning. Unless this is done, there are many cases in which, after the best management, the authority will be imperfect; and some in which any thing that deserves that name will be impossible. There are some families, not contemptible either in station or character, in which the parents are literally obedient to their children, are forced to do things against their will, and chidden if they discover the least backwardness to comply. If you know none such, I am sure I do."

CHAPTER V.

THE BEST MEANS OF PRESERVING AUTHORITY.

The Doctor's reflections on this subject are so correct, they correspond so accurately with my own observation and experience, that I cannot deny myself the pleasure of continuing the quotation, although it has already filled up three chapters. This I do the more readily having conviction that the works from which these observations are taken are not in general use in any of the southern states.

"Whatever authority you exercise over either children or servants, or as a magistrate over other citizens, it ought to be dictated by conscience, and directed by a sense of duty. Passion or resentment ought to have as little place as possible; or rather to speak properly, though few can boast of having arrived at full perfection, it ought to have no place at all. Reproof or correction given in a rage, is always considered by him to whom it is administered, as the effect of weakness in you, and therefore the demerit of the offence will be either wholly denied or soon forgotten. I have heard some parents often say, that they cannot correct their children unless they are angry; to which I have usually answered, then you ought not to correct them at all. Every one would be sensible, that for a magistrate to discover an intemperate rage in pronouncing sentence against a criminal, would be highly indecent. Ought not parents to punish their children in the same dispassionate manner? Ought they not to be at least equally concerned to discharge their duty in the best manner as well in the one case as in the other?

He who would preserve his authority over his children, should be particularly watchful of his own conduct. You may as well pretend to force people to love what is not amiable, as to reverence what is not respectable. A decency of conduct therefore, and dignity of deportment, is highly serviceable for the purpose we have now in view. Least this, however, should be mistaken, I must put in a caution, that I do not mean to recommend keeping children at too great a distance, by an uniform sternness and severity of carriage. This, I think, is not necessary, even when they are young; and to children of some tempers, it may be very hurtful when they are old. But by dignity of carriage, I mean parents always shewing themselves to be cool and reasonable in their own conduct; prudent and cautious in their conversation with regard to the rest of mankind: not fretful or impatient, or passionately fond of their own peculiarities; and though gentle and affectionate to their children, yet avoiding levity in their presence. I would have them cheerful yet serene. Their familiarity should be evidently an act of condescension. That which begets esteem will not fail to produce subjection. Every expression of affection and kindness to children is proper when it is safe, that is to say, when their behavour is such as to deserve it. There is no opposition at all between parental tenderness and parental authority. They are the best supports to each other. It is not only lawful but will be of service that parents should discover the greatest fondness for their children in infancy, and make them perceive distinctly with how much pleasure they gratify all their innocent inclinations. This however must always be done when they are quiet, gentle, and submissive in their carriage.— Some have found fault with giving them, for doing well, little rewards of sweet meats and play things, as tending to make them mercenary, & . this is refining too much.— Th great point is, that they be rewarded for doing good, and not for doing evil. When they are cross and froward, I would never buy peace, but force it. Nothing can be more weak and foolish or more destructive of authority, than when children are noisy and in an ill humour, to give them or promise them something to appease them.— When the Roman emperors began to give pensions and subsidies to the northern nations to keep them quiet, a man might have foreseen without the spirit of prophecy, who would be master in a little time. The case is exactly the same with children; they will soon avail themselves of this easiness in their parents, command favours instead of begging them, and be insolent when they should be thankful.

"The same conduct ought to be uniformly preserved as children advance in understanding. Let parents try to convince them how much they have their real interest at heart.—Sometimes children will make a request, and receive a hasty or forward denial; yet upon reflection, the thing appears not to be unreasonable, and finally it is granted, and whether it be right or wrong, sometimes by the force of importunity, it is extorted. If parents expect either gratitude or submission for favours so ungraciously bestowed, they will find themselves egregiously mistaken.—It is their duty to prosecute, and it ought to be their comfort to see the happiness of their children; and therefore they ought to lay it down as a rule, never to give a sudden or hasty refusal; but when any thing is proposed to them, consider deliberately and fully whether it is proper; and after that, either grant it cheerfully or deny it firmly.

CHAPTER VI.

PROPRIETY OF INCULCATING RELIGIOUS SENTIMENT.

"The only foundation for a useful education in a republic is to be laid in religion.—Without this there can be no virtue, and without virtue there can be no liberty, and liberty is the object and life of all republican governments."

These reflections taken from Dr. Rush's essay *on the mode of education proper in a republic*, are completely correspondent with my first fundamental proposition, Part I. chap. 2. And this excellent writer still proceeds to support my theory. "Such (says he) is my veneration for every religion that reveals the attributes of the deity, or a future state of rewards and punishments, that I had rather see the opinions of Confucius or Mahomet inculcated upon our youth, than see them grow up wholly devoid of a system of religious principles. But the religion I mean to recommend, is that of the New-Testament."

"It is foreign to my purpose to hint at the arguments which establish the truth of the Christian revelation. My only business is to declare, that all its doctrines and precepts are calculated to promote the happiness of society, and the safety and well being of civil government. A christian cannot fail of being a republican. The history of the creation of man, and of the relation of our species to each other by birth, which is recorded in the old Testament, is the best refutation that can be given to the divine right of kings, and the strongest argument that can be used in favor of the original and natural equality of all mankind. A christian I say again, cannot fail of being a republican, for every precept of the gospel inculcates those degrees of humility, self denial, and brotherly kindness, which are directly opposed to the pride of monarchy and the pageantry of a court. A christain cannot fail of being useful to the republic, for his religion teacheth him, that no man liveth to himself. And lastly, a christian cannot fail of being wholly inoffensive, for his religion teacheth him in all things to do to others what he would wish, in like circumstances, they should do to him."

"I am aware that I dissent from one of those paradoxical opinions with which modern times abound, that it is improper to fill the minds of youth with religious prejudices of any kind, and that they should be left to choose their own principles, after they have arrived at an age in which they are capable of judging for themselves., Could we preserve the mind in childhood and youth a perfect blank, this plan of education would have more to recommend it, but this we know to be impossible. The human mind runs as naturally into principles, as it does after facts; it submits with difficulty to those restraints or partial discoveries which are imposed upon it in the infancy of reason. Hence the impatience of children to be informed upon all subjects that relate to the invisible world. But I beg leave to ask, why should we pursue a different plan of education with respect to religion, from that which we pursue in teaching the arts and sciences? Do we leave our youth to acquire systems of geography, philosophy or politics, till they have arrived at an age in which they are capable of judging for themselves? We do not. I claim no more then for religion, than for the other sciences, and I add further, that if our youth are disposed, after they are of age, to think for themselves, a knowledge of one system will be the best means of conducting them in a free enquiry into other systems of religion, just as an acquaintance with one system of philosophy is the best introduction to the study of all the other systems in the world."

When we still add to the above forcible reflections, the well known fact that those children who are brought up without religious sentiment, readily become extremely licentious and fall into every kind of dissipation, the candid reader must grant that parents ought by all means to bring up their children in the fear of God.

CHAPTER VII.

HOW RELIGIOUS SENTIMENT MAY BE EXCITED IN THE MINDS OF CHILDREN MOST SUCCESSFULLY.

There are two methods of exciting religious sentiment in the minds of children.

One is direct and will include all particular instruction given for that express purpose.

The other is indirect having reference to the influence of example.

1. What kind of instruction should be *directly* employed, has been a matter of controversy. I shall wave all disputation and offer a few reflections which to me seem to be correct.

The first thing necessary to be taught is the *simple existence of a* God. The curiosity of children will prepare the way for securing this fundamental point. But before I proceed further, let me remove an objection.

It is alledged by some that children receive any kind of information more readily than that pertaining to religion. If we attempt to teach an infant, the deep mysteries of those scholastic systems, which cannot be understood even by those who teach them, it is no wonder the little pupil should express uneasiness, or even disgust. The defect is in the mode of tuition, not in the child.—The case would be very different if simple facts only were properly presented to his mind. The curiosity of children is ever awake, they are all athirst for knowledge.—They quickly discover the relation of cause and effect, and eagerly enquire "Who made it? Whence came it? &c. &c." and not perceiving the necessity of granting a FIRST CAUSE, on hearing the existence of many things ascribed to the creating power of God, they ask with equal simplicity, who made HIM? Let them be encouraged in their enquiries, and you may very quickly teach them this great truth, "*That God is.*"

But it will be a matter of small moment to teach a child the existence of Deity, unless he be also taught more or less of the divine character. And even this may be done more readily than could be expected by any who never made the trial.

What may be the essential character of an *omnipotent*, *omnipresent*, and *eternal Being*, taken in the abstract, we cannot, need not know. We are not endowed with powers to contemplate it. We are chiefly interested in the communicable and moral perfections of God; his *Holiness*, *justice*, *goodness*, *truth*, *and mercy*.

It should be remembered however, that the *incomprehensible Wisdom* and *awful Power* of God, should be employed to excite that sense of *profound veneration* which must precede all other genuine religious sentiment.

Now I believe that God made man expressly that HE might manifest HIMSELF to him, and that man might be hapyy in the enjoyment of the manifestation. We are told in scripture that "God made man in his own image," by which I would understand, *a certain power of perceiving* the beauty of Holiness—justice, goodness, truth, &c. while the perception is attended with certain emotions, highly pleasurable and improving to the person favoured with it. Perhaps in a state of original rectitude, man was blessed with this glorious perception continually, and of course the consequent emotions were continually and perfectly enjoyed by him. But since the admission of iniquity into the world, mankind are barely susceptible of this happy condition, and to attain to it, must submit to very particular discipline. There are however strings in the human heart which when properly struck will accord to these divine perfections.

We are conscious of certain pleasurable emotions on beholding *stupendous greatness*, or *superlative excellence*. We have other agreeable sensations in *performing acts of goodness*, *truth*, or *mercy*, or in seeing them performed by others. To be more particular, if we behold a man of superior dignity we feel *respect*, or *reverence*. The sensation is sublime and pleasing. An act of justice meets our approbation, and while we contemplate it with pleasure, a resolution is formed in our minds, on every similar occasion to imitate it. So likewise acts of benevolence, truth, &c. excite in us similar and correspondent emotions which afford pleasure and form the mind for similar acts. It is by a certain affinity of this kind that a proper view of the divine character excites in us the " Divine affections of *Reverence*, *Gratitude*, *Love*, *Obedience*, and *Resignation*."

The character of *Deity* is unfolded to our view by various means. " The heavens declare the glory of God and the earth is filled with his wonderful works." Objects great and small every where present themselves, challenging us as rational creatures, to trace out the perfections of the great author of all. Each discovery brings new delight, whilst it makes better the heart "of him who hath pleasure therein." This employment constitutes the most rational and sublime happiness and this I venture to affirm is the great end for which man was created.

Having taught our children the existence of a Great First Cause; we cannot begin too early to turn their attention to such displays of the divine character as they may be able to comprehend. And we should remember that every attempt in which we fail to excite some one or more of the proper affections is labour lost. Therefore when we shew them the heavens, the sun, moon and stars which God hath ordained, we should make such remarks as may inspire them with *Reverence.*

Whenever we may perceive they are particularly gratified with some article of food, we should make mention of the great *Goodness* of HIM who is the giver of all our comforts. This method would excite their *Gratitude.* As their minds expand we should call their attention to the kind interposition of providence in giving them parents, friends, houses, fields, fruit trees, beasts of burthen, and the like. Instruction given in this way will be effectual and lasting. And thus the whole course of natural history might be employed to extend their knowledge of things, and to point out to them the harmonies which are displayed throughout the works of creation, forming an infinite variety of melodious voices singing the *Wisdom*, *Power* and *Goodness* of God. Their gratitude will insensibly be mingled with *Love*, and they will be delighted with our instructions while they learn to contemplate their Creator as their great and loving Father. Their obedience to us when made habitual, and their confidence in our friendship and protection, may be employed to teach them divine Obedience and Trust. At length from a general admiration and esteem of the divine communicable perfections, they will be prepared with joy to "behold the glory of God in the face of Jesus Christ in whom dwells the fulnesss of the Godhead bodily," and by the contemplation of the character of God as there more clearly and interestingly *revealed*, be changed into the same image from glory to glory.—Let sceptics smile or approve, I am happy to declare that such a manifestation of Deity is worth an empire.

Before I leave this part of the subject let me observe, that, although children should never be confined long to any kind of religious instruction unless they express a manifest willingness for it, yet parents should daily read in their hearing a portion of scripture, chosen where it is most easily understood. And after they are old enough they should be made to read a chapter or two every day themselves. But they ought not to be compelled to pore over it till they feel disgust at the book and all those who bind them in such heavy chains.

2. It remains that something be said of the second or indirect mode of exciting religious sentiment.

The plan I recommend, requires judgment, reflection, and great attention in our whole conduct. Nothing should be admitted in the intervals that may counteract it. There should be no opposition between our precepts and examples.

As we would inculcate upon them *Reverence* to God, gravity should continually appear in our deportment. No foolish levity should be indulged. No irreverent expression should ever escape from our lips.

As we wish to inspire them with *Gratitude*, with never failing regularity we should express our thanks to God at every meal, and with the return of morning and evening assemble our children and servants for family worship.

As we desire they should imitate the Deity in *Benevolence*, we should treat all men with gentleness and kindness. We should never be guilty of "that common but detestable custom, of receiving persons with courtesy and all the marks of real friendship in our houses, and the moment they are gone, falling upon their character with unmerciful severity." We should never abuse a servant or any of our domestics, but at all times shew respect to their merit and endeavour to make them happy. We should not suffer a horse or ox to be unnecessarily tortured. We should not even approve the death of an harmless insect.

As we would have them distinguished for love of virtue, we should always pay the greatest attention to the man of real worth, without regard to the extent of his possessions. We should never seem to be gratified with a visit from the wealthy, making every possible exertion to accommodate them, when at the same time, we would scarcely treat a man in poorer circumstances with common civility.

As we would wish them to have a true knowledge of God as manifested through Christ Jesus, we should strive to be like this Divine Teacher ; *meek*, *humble*, *patient*, *long suffering*, *benevolent*, *&c. &c.*

CHAPTER VIII.

COMMON COUNTRY SCHOOLS INJURIOUS.

By the greatest attention parents form their children to virtue and religion. But it is a lamentable truth that too many entirely neglect this important duty. Most children grow up like the " wild asses' colt." This being the case it follows, that a school made up of twenty or thirty children taken promiscuously from the whole neighbourhood, is an assemblage of vice sufficient to ruin the whole. Each one is contaminated with the vices of all the rest, and so our children bad enough at best, become twenty times worse.

The person who is placed at their head is commonly some ignorant and lazy fellow, who is as little anxious as he is qualified to preserve their morals. It is true the man can read and write, and by dint of severe correction, and at the expence of a thousand helpless tears, his scholars receive a sketch of his *mighty acquirements*. Corrupted by their school-fellows, debased by their teacher's ill manners and discipline, their little stock of literature is purchased at an expence which the most liberal tour of science could not compensate.

Parents, particularly mothers, should teach their children these first rudiments of literature. Where this is impracticable, they should employ some proper person to teach them under their own inspection. Perhaps a female teacher might be preferred for several of the first years.

In neighbourhoods where the circumstances of the people make common schools necessary, the greatest care should be taken to employ the best men to teach them. It is unpardonable to prefer a worthless creature before a man of talent and worth for the sake of saving three or four dollars per year.

I shall conclude this chapter with an earnest request of all parents to educate their daughters specially. This will be doing the greatest benefit to the rising generation.—Nothing could be more important. *If it could be at once universal it would reform nations.* See Part I. Introduction.*

---

* Since the publication of this work, from some cause, the spirit of female education is diffusing itself through the state of Virginia, to an extent far surpassing any thing heretofore known. It is sincerely to be hoped, so laudable a design will never more be abandoned or neglected.

CHAPTER IX.

INTRODUCTORY REMARKS ON THE MODE OF PRESERVING THE HEALTH OF CHILDREN.

The principal things to be regarded for the preservation of the health of children are, cleanliness, liberty, free air, regular cloathing and proper food.

1. When I recommend *cleanliness*, I do not mean that they should always appear in a dress fit for seeing company ; or, that they should never be suffered to foul their hands and feet. All that can be requisite is, that they should be clean dressed once, or if convenient, twice a week. That they should lie upon clean and dry beds.* This is an important precaution, as they would receive less injury by being exposed a whole day to very inclement weather, if kept in constant action, than from lying a few hours on a wet or damp sheet. And lastly, that their skin be frequently washed with cool water. Perhaps it might be a very convenient and proper method, to change the linnen of very dirty children every night, giving them a clean and dry shirt to sleep in, and in the morn-

* There are some people who do not expose their beds to the sun as often as they ought; this should be done twice a week.

ing putting on again the clothes in which they may be suffered to roll about in the dirt.*

2. By recommending *liberty*, I intend to speak against the improper custom of keeping children too much confined in the arms of their nurse, and of shutting them up in any one particular apartment. They should be indulged in running about the house or yard at will. Care should be taken however, that they do not climb upon dangerous places. In this respect, the greatest latitude may be given them, and yet with a very little attention, the thing might be so conducted, as in a gradual and unperceived manner, to lay the foundation for their future regularity and industry; but they should never be left in the

* There are some who through ignorance of its ill effects, or through the most inexcusable indolence, suffer little ponds of water and filth to stand in their yards or under their houses for months together.—Such will probably pay very dearly for their want of cleanliness. I have seen some which might ultimately produce the most maglignant diseases.

Not intending by any means to insult the feelings of the ladies, it is presumed the better informed will thank me for stating the impropriety and scandal of permitting *loathsome insects* so to infest houses and beds, that people of taste and decency cannot rest in them It is hoped that *all* American women will shun such a disgrace by paying proper attention to that neatness for which *many, very many* of them already deserve the highest credit.

care of a heedless or vicious nurse; for in such hands, not only their lives are in danger, but they learn habits which may be pernicious to their morals and happiness through life. This last precaution well deserves the attention of the rich. They too often give up the management of their children to ignorant and immoral slaves, whose interest it is to contaminate the minds of their little masters, that through them they may in future obtain favours and indulgencies.

3. Sufficient liberty being granted them, they will of course breathe in a pure and *free air* during the day. But I must here make a remark on the danger of putting children to sleep in a close room, from which every breath of air is excluded. Many promising children have perished in convulsions, by this act of mistaken kindness.

4. As to the *cloathing* of children, it is important that every part of it be made loose and easy. Confinement in this respect must endanger their health by obstructing the regular motions of the system, and may at length deform them very much. Their dress should be moderately warm, and should be varied with the weather and seasons. It will be found on observation, that in most instances *violent fever* and *croup* happen to those children who are most healthy, and who of

course are pemitted to run about in cold and windy weather without any change of cloathing. A very moderate degree of care on the part of the mother might prevent much mischief in this respect.

5. In the article of food, children may generally be permitted to indulge their own appetite. If healthy, they will eat more or less for every hour in the day. It is much better for their health to gratify them as often as they request it, than to confine them to any set meals adapted to the demands of grown people.

While they are young, milk is the best, and ought to be a principal article of their food. "*Milk* (says Dr. Darwin) is the natural food for children, and must curdle in their stomachs before digestion ; and as this curdling of the milk destroys a part of the acid juices of the stomach, there is no reason for discontinuing its use, although it is occasionally thrown out in a curdled state. A child of a week old, which had been taken from the breast of its dying mother, and by some uncommon error, had been suffered to take no food but water gruel, became sick and griped in twenty-four hours, was convulsed on the second day, and died on the third. When young children are brought up without a breast, for the first two months they should have no food but new milk." It should be weakened with a little water, and some loaf or clean brown sugar, might also be added. But "the addition of any kind of bread or flour is liable to ferment and produce much acidity; as appears by the consequent diarrhœa with green stools and gripes. And they should never be fed as they lie upon their backs, as in that position they are necessiated to swallow all that is put into their mouths; but when they are fed as they are sitting up, or raised pretty much, when they have had enough, they can permit the rest to run out of their mouths. This circumstance is of great importance to the health of those children who are reared by the spoon, since if too much food is given them, indigestion, gripes and diarrhoea, are the consequences; and if too little, they become emaciated; and of the exact quantity, their own palates judge the best."

Most mothers from their natural tenderness for their infant children, are led to feed them more or less of every article of which they eat themselves. In some instances it may not happen to do any mischief. But it is always dangerous to oppose the obvious appointments of the God of nature. If we would be guided by the intimations given us of his *will*, we should never feed our children with solid food, till they were supplied with teeth for masticating it. I think no vegitable should be given them till they are at least five months old.

CHAPTER X.

SOME REMARKS, INTRODUCTORY TO THE CURE OF THE COMMON DISEASES INCIDENT TO CHILDREN.

It is common for parents to be wholly dependent on physicians, for the relief of their children whenever they are sick. In difficult and dangerous cases, it certainly it best to procure the most judicious advice. But as no one can be so deeply interested in the health and happiness of their children as the parents themselves, it follows, if they have the necessary information, that they must be the proper persons to prescribe to their complaints. The truth of this may perhaps hereafter appear. If parents could know the symptoms which usher in a violent attack of fever, by being continually with their children, they might always be apprized of their first disposition to disease. This circumstance would be very important since a disease of whatever kind, is most easily removed in its forming state. Nay more, a very simple system of medical knowledge would answer this intention. Such an one, as any person of common understanding might execute. But a fixed disease is ever difficult of management, and may not only perplex but baffle the most skilful physician. Besides there are diseases which require immediate assistance. The croup for example, frequently carries off the patient so speedily, as not even to admit of calling in a physician from the distance of one mile.

To prepare the heads of families for this important trust, would indeed be a great performance. It may not be accomplished in half a century. But every attempt, however feeble, if well directed to this great end, demands the attention and gratitude of the public.

CHAPTER XI.

SOME HINTS TO ENABLE PARENTS TO DETERMINE WHETHER THEIR CHILDREN ARE PARTICULARLY SUBJECT TO DISEASE, AND IF DISORDERED, TO JUDGE OF THE VIOLENCE OF THE ATTACK.

Parents should be particularly attentive to observe their children minutely in all their actions and habits, &c.

1. They should observe the common extent of their appetite, so that any considerable excess or deficiency in their eating may not pass unnoticed. This will be of use, since a considerable change in one of these respects, almost always takes place before a spell of sickness.

2. Attention should be paid to their stools. Unimportant as this might at first appear to the inconsiderate, yet a costive habit generally precedes an attack of fever.

3. The degree of exercise and the agility with which it is performed deserve particular observation. For all fevers are ushered in with a degree of slothfulness, a sense of weariness, and in children with a more than usual disposition to sleepiness.

4. By noticing whether any of the foregoing circumstances take place after having been exposed to unusual weather, or to greater than ordinary fatigue : Or if the place or season be sickly, by having regard to these circumstances, there will be the less danger of being taken at surprize.

5. As it is generally the case that some complaints of lesser magnitude go before and give warning of the impending danger ; such as *costiveness*, a *sense of weariness*, *dullness of the faculties*, *preternatural appetite or defect of it*, *a pain in the limbs*, &c. There-

fore when these marks of forming disease present themselves, a puke or purge ought to be timely administered according to circumstances. This might frequently prevent great mischief. Indeed in many instances, simply bathing the feet in hot water, and taking a plentiful draught of warm tea of some kind on going to bed, might prevent an attack of fever, especially if the patient be not in a costive habit. This last circumstance may be considered in most instances as requiring the exhibition of a purge of some kind. As also great sickness of the stomach might point out the propriety of a puke.

6. But it will also be important for parents to be able to judge of the violence of the disease in case of an attack. They should therefore frequently observe the strength of their children's pulse when in health, *its kind of motion*, the *force with which it seems to propel the blood* along, *its apparent size*, *its tightness as to its extension lengthwise of the arm*, *its fulness*, &c. A knowledge of these circumstances attending the pulse, will be very important in particular cases, especially where bleeding may be necessary. For this operation cannot be proper unless the pulse be either strong and full, or *tight*, at least judicious advice should be had in cases with other states of the pulse.

7. They should also have regard to the manner of breathing in a healthy child, to the state of his skin, the appearance of his eyes, the complexion of his teeth, the colour and degree of moisture of his tongue, the proper figure and appearance of his mouth and throat. For as the violence and danger of a disease are always in proportion to the irregularity presented in these circumstances and appearances, it must be important to obtain a correct knowledge of them all.

8. Let us apply these remarks in a case or two. It may be observed that children are subject to some of the most violent diseases. If a child after exposure to cold, be taken suddenly at night when warm in bed, if the pulse be strong, full and tight, if it beat forcibly in the neck, if the face be flushed with blood, while there is great heat and thirst, if he breathe irregularly, with a stoppage at every breath, if he have a cough, and particularly if he express an increase of pain on pressing his side with the hand, a *pleurisy* should be suspected, and he should be immediately bled; and this operation should be repeated again and again, as often as the violence of the symptoms require it. A large bleeding at the first is better than smaller ones repeated. It should be so large as at any rate to change the manner of his breath-

ing and lessen the pain. The blood should be drawn from a large orifice. After a copious bleeding, let three grains of tartar emetic and twenty grains of salt petre* be dissolved in one gill of water, and give a tea-spoonful of this solution in barley water, or flax-seed tea, or any other mild drink a little warmed, every one two or three hours. It will moderate the cough and remove the fever. If it nauseate too much, the dose should be lessened. As this calculation would suit a child of four or five years old, the quantity of tartar should be varied according to circumstances. In the mean time his bowels should be evacuated with a little manna, cream of tartar, castor oil, or some other mild purge. Glysters might also be of service.

9. Again, if the child complain of pain in the head, attended with redness of the eyes and face. If the admission of the light to his eyes seem to excite uneasiness or pain, if he startle at every noise, be very watchful sometimes making violent struggles, and have a full and tight, or hard pulse, *inflammation of the brain* should be suspected.—In this case the child should be copiously

* The salt petre if rejected by the patient, might be left out of the solution.

bled, purged with jalap and calomel, and glystered. His head should be considerably raised, cloths wet with cold water and vinegar should be applied to his head, and after bleeding and purging for four or five days, a blister should be applied to his head (shaved for the purpose) or to his two temples.

10. I have introduced the above cases in this place, because more or less of those symptoms indicating danger to the *lungs* and *brain*, frequently occur in measles, whooping cough, and other diseases of children ; and because it is important that these parts of the system so essential to life, should be properly guarded whatever may be the supposed complaint. Whether it may be owing to the greater proportionate size of the *head*, and the more delicate contexture of the *lungs* in children, or to whatever cause it may be referred, it is a fact, that in all fevers there is a greater determination of the blood to the brain and lungs in children's cases than in those of adults.

CHAPTER XII.

RED GUM.

I now proceed to consider some of the particular diseases to which children are exposed. And the first to be noticed is commonly called *Red Gum;* it has its name from its appearance, being a red eruption on any part of the body or face of very young children; it is is not dangerous, and generally goes off in a few days. Dr. Darwin supposes it may be the effect of heat, and the friction of flannel.

CHAPTER XIII.

JAW FALL.

Another disease of young children is the *Jaw Fall;* the name is sufficiently expressive of its nature. I think it seldom occurs in this country. And whenever it does happen, it is said to be incurable. It may be prevented however, by purging the child soon after its birth with the following preparation. Take magnesia twenty grains, rhubarb five grains, grind them carefully together. Of this powder give from three to five grains every four or six hours, till the evacuations are sufficiently copious. Some think this an excellent remedy and recommend it in all cases of new born children. Perhaps it would seldom be improper where the natural discharges are deficient. It may be given in a little breast milk or fennel seed tea with or without sugar.

CHAPTER XIV.

SORE OR RUPTURED NAVEL.

If the child be distressed with a sore navel, mix together ten grains of the sugar of lead and forty grains of wheat flour. Sprinkle the sore with this powder twice or three times a day, after having each time cleansed it carefully and tenderly with milk and water. Cotton or lint scorched very brown will commonly dry up the sore speedily after the redness is removed by using the above powder, or by the application of the bread and milk poultice. Borax dissolved in water is sometimes proper.

For a ruptured navel apply a plaister made of the diachylon salve and common resin ; say diachylon five parts, resin one part to be melted together. This application acts merely by confining the istestine to its proper place till nature may have time to perform the cure.

CHAPTER XV.

THRUSH.

This is a very common complaint among young children. Its first approach may be known by sleepiness, and might generally be prevented by a few doses of the powder recommended in chap. XIII. When this disease takes place, the tongue becomes in some degree swelled. Its colour and that of the throat is purplish. Sloughs or rather ulcers appear, first on the throat and edges of the tongue, and at length over the whole mouth. These sloughs or ulcers are of a whitish colour, sometimes they are quite distinct and in some instances run together. The time of its duration is uncertain.

For the cure let the mouth be carefully and gently washed several times in the day with the following solution. To half a gill of water well sweetened with molasses or honey, add fifteen grains of borax. When dissolved it is ready for use. Or if this should not be convenient, take sage tea half a gill sweetened as before, add to it from five to ten grains of the best almond soup, to be used in the same manner as the former.

CHAPTER XVI.

MILK IN THE BREASTS.

It is very common for milk to collect in young childrens breasts, and their nurses intending them a kindness, cruelly squeese it out by dint of force. This should never be done, because it sometimes induces a hard and dangerous swelling. The milk may be scattered by bathing the breasts with a little spirit, or by applying an ointment made of oil and camphire.

CHAPTER XVII.

BELLY-ACHE.

This complaint is commonly the consequence either of the mother's eating too much rich food, or of feeding the child too soon on vegetable diet. Women giving such should prefer a vegetable diet. Milk also is an excellent article for them at such times. Children should be weaned at ten or twelve months old; or at any event on the return of menstruation. The remedies proper for the belly-ache are peppermint water, tincture of opium or paregoric elixir, or the powder recommended in chap. XIII. but spirits should never be used. If tincture of opium be chosen for the purpose, not more than one fourth part of a drop ought to be given for the first dose, but it may afterwards be repeated and gradually enlarged. I have known a child of two weeks old to be convulsed from taking one drop at once.

I will conclude this chapter with observing that no disease can be communicated from the mother to the child through the channel of her milk.

CHAPTER XVIII.

TEETHING.

Children seldom begin to cut their teeth till they are three months old, and some not till they are much older. The symptoms are, a *vomiting*, *lax*, *fever*, *starting-fits*, *swelled and sore ears*, and *swelling* of the *glands* or *kernels* of the *throat* and *groins*. The remedies are cold air, tincture of opium and finally cutting the gums. They should be cut lengthwise in the direction of the gums, and quite through to the bone; but if it be thought more convenient they may be cut across.

CHAPTER XIX.

ERUPTIONS ON THE SKIN.

Where considerable eruptions break out upon the skin of children in other respects quite healthy, and of a full habit, their nurse should live upon a vegetable diet, and the child should be purged; for this purpose nothing perhaps is better than calomel. A child of three months old, might take from half a grain to a grain; of six months old, from one to two grains; of nine months up to a year, from one to three grains.

If the eruptions happen to a weakly and delicate child, let the nurse eat more generous food, &c.

CHAPTER XX.

WARTS ON THE TONGUE; TONGUE TIED; COSTIVENESS.

Warts on the tongue may be clipped with a very sharp pair of scissors. Where the tongue is tied, the frenum or string under the tongue may be divided with the same instrument; and it is always best to do it while the child is young.

Costiveness may be corrected with the powder recommended in chap. XIII. or with castor oil, manna, or the like.

CHAPTER XXI.

FALLING DOWN OF THE LOWER INTESTINE.

Children who cry much, or are long under the influence of a diarrhoea, are subject to the falling down of the straight gut. We are told of various means for preventing it. The following is perhaps as good as any.

If the gut be considerably protruded, swelled and inflamed, let it be well bathed with warm milk and water, and then let a large and soft poultice of bread and milk be applied, to be exchanged for a fresh one every three or four hours till the inflammation is removed. Should the swelling and inflammation be so obstinate as not to yield to this method, let the part be well scarified so as to evacuate the blood freely. Then apply the poultice as before and give the patient a dose of the tincture of opium. The scarifications, poultices, &c. should be repeated till the gut can be readily replaced. Then having washed it with a decoction of oak bark let it be returned and kept up by the aid of a bandage or truss; and this should be done after every stool if the descent of the intestine should make it necessary. In the mean time a costive habit must be carefully prevented by the use of small doses of castor oil or some other gentle purge.

CHAPTER XXII

WORMS.

The most learned physicians are of opinion that there is no such a disease as a *worm-fever*, and that the disease erroneously known by that name is an *internal dropsy of the brain.*

The symptoms pointing out the presence of worms are various and are the following: Grinding of the teeth, starting in sleep, dry cough bringing up a frothy spittle, sighing and suffocating manner of breathing, pain in the side, hiccup, heart-burn, vomiting, lax, sudden urgings to go to stool, costiveness, slimy stools, night sweats, sour breath, flushing of one cheek, itching of the nose, an excessive appetite, lying much on the belly, swelling of the partition of the nose and of the upper lip, the actual voiding of more or less worms, a wasting away of the limbs and of the whole body, jaundice, head-ache, deadly snoring in sleep, convulsions, &c. &c.

Our first care should be to prevent the dangerous effects of worms, and there are various articles of food which will answer this intention. "Nature" says Dr. Rush in his medical enquiries "has wisely guarded children against the morbid effects of worms by implanting in them an early appetite for *common salt*, *ripe fruits* and saccharine substances, all of which appear to be among the most speedy and effectual poisons for worms. Ever since I observed the effects of *sugar* and other *sweet substances* upon worms, I have recommended the liberal use of all of them in the diet of children with the happiest effects."

The medicines proper for the removal of worms are.

1. Common salt; this may be given in doses of thirty grains upon an empty stomach in the morning, and is an excellent remedy.

2. Sugar or molasses in large quantities, so that they may pass out of the stomach without undergoing any material change from digestion. In smaller quantities they will destroy worms in the stomach only.

3. The expressed juice of onions and garlic are said to be considerably efficacious against the excess of worms.

4. Gun-powder; a tea spoonful to be given in the morning upon an empty stomach. Perhaps three fourths of the same quantity of salt petre would answer just as well.

5. Carolina pink root; if this article be properly used it is a very certain remedy. About half an ounce may be gently stewed in half a pint of water till its strength is pro-

perly extracted. Then let the decoction be strained and well sweetened with sugar or molasses, and give one fourth of it every two or three hours to a child four or five years old. I have generally thought it best to add to each dose about one eighth of an ounce of manna. The importance of this addition will appear when it is remembered that, the pink root is poisonous and if given in too large quantities kills the child to whom it is given.

6. Aloes, four to six grains, rhubarb eight to fifteen grains, Jesuits bark, bears-foot, worm-seed, these are all said to be good *worm medicines*.

7. Calomel; this is an excellent and safe remedy whether given by itself or combined with jalap. It is most effectual however when given in large doses, from four to eight grains might be given to a child of four to six years old.

8. "But of all the medicines that I have administered," says Dr. Rush, "I know of none more safe and certain than the simple preparations of *iron*, whether they be given in the form of *steel-filings*, or of *rust of iron*. If ever they fail of success, it is because they are given in too small doses. I generally prescribe from five to thirty grains every morning, to children between one and ten

years old; and I have been taught by an old sea captain, who was cured of a *tape worm* by this medicine to give from two drams to half an ounce of it every morning, for three or four days not only with safety but with success."

CHAPTER XXIII.

INTERNAL DROPSY OF THE BRAIN.

This disorder is sometimes the consequence of a stroke upon the head received by falling or otherwise. It may also be excited by different kinds of fever.

In every case where there are pains of the limbs and head, sickness at the stomach, dilatation of one or both pupils of the eyes, and sleepiness, this disease should be suspected.

Dr. Rush in treating of this complaint in his enquiries gives the following description of it as taken from the writings of Dr. Quin.

" In general the patient is at first languid " and inactive, often drowsy and peevish " but at intervals cheerful and apparently " free from complaint. The appetite is " weak, and in many cases a vomiting occurs

" once or twice in the day, and the skin is " observed to be hot and dry towards the " evening. Soon after these symptoms " have appeared, the patient is affected with " a sharp headache, chiefly in the fore part, " and if not there generally in the crown of " the head. It is sometimes however con- " fined to one side of the head, and in that " case, when the posture of the body is erect, " (as in sitting,) the head often inclines to " the side affected." The vomiting is less troublesome when the pain in the head is most violent, and the contrary. There are also pains in the limbs or the bowels, but more constantly in the back of the neck and between the shoulder blades; and in these cases the head is commonly less affected.

" The patient dislikes the light at this pe- " riod, cries much, sleeps little, and when he " does sleep he grinds his teeth, picks his " nose, appears to be uneasy, and starts often, " screaming as if he were terrified." The bowels are in most cases bound, though sometimes they are in a lax state ; and the pulse is not much irregular in this early stage of the disorder.*

* I take the liberty sometimes to abridge Dr. Quin's history and state it in a language more plain and easy for common readers.

"These symptoms are subject to great fluctuation, but whatever may be the degree or order of them, after some days one of the eyes will be turned inwards as if looking at the nose, and the pupil of the turned eye will be more dilated than the other; and if both eyes be turned which sometimes happens, both pupils will be larger than they are observed to be in healthy people at the same time, and in the same degree of light. After this the vomiting becomes more constant, and the head-ache more excruciating; every symptom of fever makes its appearance; the pulse is frequent, the breathing quick; the fever returns with more violence at night, and the face is flushed; usually one cheek more than the other. There are temporary sweats and sometimes bleeding at the nose, but neither affords any relief. The patient is sometimes violently delirious."

"After proceeding on in this way for fourteen days, often a much shorter space of time, the disorder undergoes a change and passes into the second stage. The pulse becomes slow and unequal both in time and strength, the pains seem to abate, a deep sleepiness ensues, the pupils are more dilated; the patient lies with one or both eyes half closed which are found on examination to be insensible to light; the vomiting ceases, the patient swallows with greediness whatever is offered to him, and the bowels remain obstinately costive."

"If not relieved, the second stage is soon succeeded by the third, which speedily terminates in death. The symptoms in this stage are a weak and quick but equal pulse, difficult breathing with deep snoring, the eyes suffused with blood; alternate flushings and deadly paleness of the face; red spots or blotches on the limbs, difficulty of swallowing, and lastly convulsions close the scene."

I must here observe however, that neither the dilated or insensible pupil, nor the puking, the delirium or the squinting always attend this disease. Children of every age, but more commonly those of four or five years old, are subject to it.

As was hinted before, this is the complaint which was little understood till lately, and was commonly called a *worm fever*. And as worms are in some instances discharged in this disorder, ignorant and injudicious persons may readily enough be deceived. In every instance therefore where the symptoms are suspicious, parents ought to be alarmed, and if possible, they should procure relief on the first attack.

1. The remedies to be employed in the first stage of this too often fatal disease are *bleeding* and *purging*. These should be repeated as often as may be necessary to subdue the inflammation. If there be pain in the head, cold water, or vinegar and water, or even ice-water might be applied with cloths wetted for the purpose, which should be frequently changed. Sometimes the symptoms abate after two or three bleedings, but return in the course of a few days. In every such instance the bleeding must be repeated and the more certainly so if the pulse be full and tight.

2. In the last stages of this complaint bleeding is seldom proper. The principal dependance is to be placed on the use of mercury. The patient should be salivated.

At any stage of the disease after the inflammatory symptoms are subdued, blisters are beneficial and should be applied to the head, neck, and temples.

CHAPTER XXIV.

CROUP OR HIVES.

In this disease Dr. Rush makes two important distinctions. The first is attended with spasm and a dry cough. The second is without spasm and the patient under its influence, is able to cough up a considerable quantity of phlegm.

1. The spasmodic croup comes on suddenly and that generally in the night; has frequent and perfect intermissions of the symptoms for hours and sometimes even for days, is attended with a dry cough as above, and is at last particularly relieved by the use of the warm bath, assafoetida, opium, &c. To be particular; the child will probably go to bed in good health, and in an hour or two wake in a fright with his face much flushed, or even of a purple colour, he will be unable to describe what he feels, will breathe with much labour, and with a peculiar convulsive motion of his belly; his breathing will also be very quick, attended with a sound as if he were threatened with a speedy suffocation; the terror of the child increases his disorder, and he will cling to the nurse; and if not speedily relieved by coughing, belching, sneezing, vomiting or purging, the suffocation will increase and the child will die. It is remarkable that the cough in this disease very much resembles in sound the barking of a young dog.

There are also during the continuance of the disorder, frequent eruptions of little red blotches on the skin, which for the time seem to afford relief; and this eruption will sometimes appear and disappear two or three times in the course of the complaint. For the cure in this first distinction of the croup, the remedies are,

1. Bleeding. When the difficulty of breathing is great, the face much flushed, or when the patient expresses much pain in coughing, this remedy is absolutely necessary, and should be repeated as often as may be requisite for subduing these symptoms.

2. Vomits. From five to six grains of ipecacuanha with two or three grains of calomel may be given to a child from two to four years old, or half a grain of tartar emetic with three or four grains of ipecacuanha; or five grains of ipecacuanha with two or three grains of turpeth mineral; or a teaspoonful of antimonial wine; or a spoonful of a strong decoction of seneka, called also rattle-snake root. Which ever dose is used, it should be repeated till the intended effect is produced, but bleeding ought first to be performed.

3. Purges. Jalap and calomel, from five to ten grains of the former with two or four of the latter may be given to a child of three to five years old. Or calomel alone from three to five or six grains; or jalap eight to

twelve grains; or castor oil, but this is scarcely active enough for so violent a disease.

4. Warm bath. This may be used either before or after bleeding, but it will be most effectual after the evacuations, and ought to be repeated daily for some time.

5. Glysters. Milk and water or chicken broth or thin gruel may be used for this purpose and in some instances where the spasm remains after bleeding, &c. fifteen drops of the tincture of opium may be occasionally added to the injections. Ten to fifteen grains of tartar emetic dissolved in half a pint of thin gruel or chicken water is an excellent injection.

6. Blisters will be found very serviceable after the evacuations of bleeding and purging; these may be applied to the back part of the neck or to the side of the patient.

7. When blisters are properly admissible, opium, assafoetida, &c. may be used with safety.

II. The second distinctions of this disorder is attended with symptoms very similar to those of the first, but may be known by its coming on gradually and that commonly in the day time; by its continuing and frequently increasing for several days without any remarkable remission or even abatement of the symptoms ; by the discharge of phlegm from the wind pipe by coughing, as also by the appearance of slime in the stools ; and lastly by its refusing to yield to the warm bath, opium, &c.

The remedies proper in this kind of croup are as before, but with some variation.

1. Bleeding when the breathing is difficult, the face flushed, the pulse tight, &c.

2. Vomits, as under the first distinction.

3. Purges. But in this case calomel only should be used ; the principal dependance should be placed upon this medicine. A large dose should be given as soon as the disorder discovers itself ; six or eight grains to a child four years old. Afterwards smaller doses should be given every day so long as any of the symptoms continue. From two to four grains might answer this intention.

It is important that relief should be afforded on the first attack of this violent disease. If neglected it will be fatal in almost every instance.

CHAPTER XXV.

CHOLERA MORBUS ; OR PURGING AND VOMITING.

This disorder makes its appearance in warm climates as early in the season as April and May, but in colder climates not till the middle of June or first of July.

The danger attending it is in proportion to the heat of the weather. Children are subject to it from one or two weeks till two years old.

It sometimes begins with a diarrhea, which will continue for several days without any other disorder ; but most commonly violent *vomiting* and *purging* and *high fever* attend. The matter discharged from the stomach and bowels is yellow or green, and the stools are sometimes slimsy and mixed with blood without any appearance of bile ; sometimes too the stools are thin as water ; worms are frequently voided whether the evacuations be bilious or not : the patient seems to suffer much pain ; draws up his feet and is never easy in one posture ; his pulse is weak and quick ; his head very warm while his hands and feet are cold ; the fever remits and returns with greater violence every evening ; his head is sometimes so much affected that he not only becomes delirious, but will rave and try to scratch or bite his parents or nurse ; his belly and sometimes his face and limbs swell ; he has great thirst in every stage ; his eyes appear languid and hollow and he sleeps with them half closed ; so great is the insensibility of his eyes that flies light upon them while open and do not excite the least motion in the eye-lids.

Sometimes the vomiting continues without the purging, but more commonly the purging remains without the vomiting through the whole course of the disorder.

The stools are sometimes large, emitting a very disagreeable smell; at other times there are scanty stools without smell, and like the food or drink taken in by the child.

This disorder is sometimes fatal in a few days and in some cases even in twenty-four hours. Much depends on the state of the weather, one cool day frequently abates its violence. The time of its duration varies exceedingly, from a few days to six weeks or two months. When it is of long standing and tending to death, there is commonly great wasting of the patient's flesh, his bones will sometimes come through the skin. Towards the close of the disease there appear purple spots on the skin with hiccup, convulsions, ghastly countenance and sore mouth. When these last appearances come on, the case has generally become incurable.

The following remarks may help to guard against mistakes in this disease.

1. It is sometimes thought to be the effect of teething; but as it comes on at a particular season of the year this mistake may be

avoided. It is true however that it is rendered more violent when it happens to seize upon children in the time of teething.

2. It is sometimes attributed to worms; but although worms are frequently voided in this fever they are never the cause of it.

3. It has been considered the effect of eating summer fruits; but where children can get ripe fruits at pleasure, it seldom occurs, and indeed ripe fruits taken moderately have a considerable tendency to prevent it. On the whole it may be considered a species of billious fever, and may be cured as follows;

1. Give a puke to evacuate the bile from the stomach; this may be done by the aid of a dose of ipecacuanha or tartar emetic, and it should be repeated as often as there is vomiting of bile, in every stage of the disorder.

2. The bowels should then be purged with manna, castor oil, or magnesia. Rhubarb is not a proper remedy till the fever is subdued in some considerable degree. If however the puking and purging have continued till there is good reason to believe that the offending matter has been thrown off by the natural efforts, the pukes and purges must be omitted, and instead of them,

3. A few drops of the tincture of opium may be given in a chalk julep. Say, prepared chalk or crabs claws eight grains to twenty;

tincture of opium half a drop to three or four, cinnamon water or peppermint tea at discretion; syrrup as much as may be sufficient to make it pleasant; to be given every three, four or six hours. Sometimes a few drops of spirits of hartshorn will be a useful addition to the above julep.

4. Small blisters might be applied to the region of the stomach, or to the wrists and ankles.

5. Mint and mallows teas, or blackberry briar root infused in cold water; a decoction of shavings of hartshorn; or a solution of gum arabic; or the pith of sassafras wood steeped in warm water with the addition of a little mint or cinnamon; either of these articles may be prepared and used as a drink to compose the stomach or bowels.

6. Glysters made of flax-seed tea, or of mutton broth, or of starch dissolved in water; either of these with the addition of a few drops of tincture of opium may be frequently injected.

7. Plaisters of Venice treacle where it can be had, or flannels wetted with a strong infusion of bitter herbs in warm spirits or Madeira wine, might be applied to the stomach; or what might be still more convenient, a cloth folded so as to be two or three inches

square might be wetted with the tincture of opium and applied as before.

8. As soon as the violent symptoms are subdued give bark in the form of a decoction or in substance, to which may be added a little nutmeg ; or if bark be offensive to the patient, use port wine or claret in itsstead.* At this stage it will be proper to indulge the child in any particular article of strong food he may happen to crave, as salted or dried fish, salt meat, butter or rich gravies, and even the strongest cheese.

9. Another remedy when there is great pain, is the warm bath, and it would be still more effectual if wine were used instead of water. It is also probable that a cold bath a few times repeated would be an excellent remedy.

10. In the recovering stage of the disease it will be found very beneficial to carry the child out to breathe a fresh country air.

In places where this complaint prevails, the following precautions will probably prevent it.

1. The daily use of the cold bath.

2. The dress of children should be care-

* Peruvian Bark quilted between two pieces of India cotton, and made up in the form of a waistcoat, may be worn as an excellent remedy in the last stages of the disease.

fully accommodated to the state and changes of the weather.

3. Salted meat should be daily but moderately used through the sickly season.

4. Good sound wine may be given them in portions adapted to their age; from a tea-spoonful to half a wine glass full at the discretion of their parents.

5. Particular regard should be had to cleanliness both with respect to their skin and cloathing.

6. Lastly, persons living in sickly towns ought to be specially attentive to all these precautions; and where it can be done they should remove their children to the country before the sickly season.

CHAPTER XXVI.

DYSSENTERY, OR BLOODY FLUX.

This disease is defined by Dr. Cullen, a contagious fever attended with frequent slimy or bloody stools, while at the same time the usual contents of the intestines are for the most part retained; and with a violent griping and a painful and frequent urging to go to stool. If there be a frequent desire of going to stool especially after eating or drinking, it is considered a certain mark of this disease. It occurs in the same seasons that intermittent fevers do, and like them, it follows long dry, long moist and hot weather. Sometimes it comes on with cold shiverings and other marks of fever, and in some instances the fever attending is very violent and inflammatory. Sometimes though not so frequently a diarrhoea is the first symptom. There is commonly a loss of appetite, frequent sickness, nausea, and vomiting which are considerably proportioned to the violence of the disease. In every case where there is violent fever the danger is considerable.

In the cure of this disease regard must be had to the degree of fever present, for if there be great thirst, acute pains and a tight though small pulse, the patient should be,

1. Bled ; and if the pains and other violent symptoms continue, the blood-letting must be repeated every twelve or twenty-four hours till they do yield.

2. Pukes are sometimes proper, but they should be used when there is great sickness at the stomach only, and if the marks of fever as above be present, a puke should not be administered till after one or more bleedings.

3. Purges should be frequently repeated,

but they must be of the most gentle sort, as cream of tartar, purging salts, manna, castor oil, &c. one of these should be used every day while the disease continues. Let it be remembered that jalap and rhubarb are not proper in this complaint.

4. Glysters of flax-seed tea or mutton broth with a little tincture of opium should be injected two, three or four times, for every twenty-four hours. If there be great heat and pain in the bowels cold water might be injected in the form of a glyster ; and indeed it could do no injury if there were no very inflammatory symptoms.

5. Opium. A dose of the tincture, or a pill of the solid opium should be given every night ; and after sufficient evacuations it might be used every six or eight hours if necessary.*

6. Cooling drinks. Whey, flax-seed tea, camomile tea not too strong, mallows tea, mullen tea, and barley water, are all proper for this purpose. And if there be much fever cold water is a very proper drink.

7. A decoction of gum arabic or shavings of hartshorn with spices ; mutton suet boiled in milk ; a decoction of black-berry roots, or a gruel made of a little flour prepared accor-

* Opium is seldom safely used until the patient has been sufficiently bled and purged.

ding to Dr. Buchan, viz. Take a few handfuls of fine flour, tie it up in a linnen cloth, and boil it in a pot for six hours till it becomes as hard as starch ; afterwards grate it and make it into gruel. Either of these will be very useful when the patient is much spent.

8. Blisters may be applied to the wrists and ankles, but not commonly until after the fifth day.

9. In the close of the disease, port wine, madeira or sherry wines are proper.

10. Where the fever intermits, and especially where it assumes the shape of the *third day fever and ague*, the bark is a very proper remedy, to be given chiefly in the fore part of the day.*

11. To prevent the contagion from spreading the patient should be kept very clean.—His room should be well aired and properly cleansed, and vinegar should be frequently poured upon a hot brick, stone, or piece of iron.

12. To prevent this disease, have regard to the instructions given in chap. XXV. part IV. for preventing cholera morbus.

---

* Or apply the bark-waistcoat, as advised in a note under the foregoing disease

CHAPTER XXVII.

MESENTERIC FEVER.

There is another disease which has its principal seat in the intestinal glands, and may therefore be properly enough admissible in this place. It is a fever excited by obstructions in the mesentery, from which circumstance it has its name. Children are subject to it from infancy up to the age of three or four, and even six or eight years.

This fever remits, and sometimes has irregular intermissions, is attended with loss of appetite, swelled belly and pain in the bowels, and has often been mistaken for worms. If therefore the usual remedies for worms should fail, the child will sooner or later be affected with very great indigestion; costiveness or purging; irregular appetite; flushed cheeks or total loss of colour; impaired strength and spirits; remitting fever; a hard swelled belly; and emaciated limbs. These symptoms will therefore sufficiently specify the disease.

It frequently follows measles and other eruptive fevers. Children that are confined to coarse and unwholesome food, are badly cloathed, not kept sufficiently clean, or neglected so as not to receive sufficient exercise, are most subject to its attack. Hence the negro children of the southern states frequently perish with this fever.

After this information, it is hoped, that if the humane feelings of slave-holders will not compel them to do justice to their blacks, a sense of interest will direct them to use the necessary pains for the preservation of their property.

When any symptoms of this destructive disease present themselves, enquiry should be made into the manner of feeding, cloathing and cleaning the child. Every error in these articles must be corrected.

If the patient have not too long laboured under its influence, frequent purging with calomel will of itself perform a cure.

In more advanced stages of this complaint, it would be best to call in the aid of a physician. But where this is impracticable proceed to give the following bolus three times a week. Take calomel two grains, ipecacuanha from half a grain to one grain, nutmeg or ginger powdered six grains, to be mixed up in honey or syrrup for one dose for a child from two to four years old. Fifteen or twenty drops of antimonial wine may be given the intervening nights where the calomel is not used.

Having continued these remedies till the

fever is removed, the hardness of the belly subsided, &c. then the strength of the patient should be restored by the use of bark, steel, cold bath, bitters of columbo and orange peel, or camomile flowers, &c. gentle exercise, friction, light nourishing food, &c. &c. All greasy or fat articles should be avoided, as also those preparations of pastry which are of a clammy nature.

CHAPTER XXVIII.

HOOPING COUGH.

This disease commonly falls upon a whole neighbourhood about the same time, and is therefore said to be epidemic. It is manifestly contagious, and like several other contagions, it affects persons but once in the course of their lives. Children therefore are most commonly the subjects of it. Sometimes however it occurs in persons considerably advanced in life. Grown persons and those who are elderly, in proportion to their age, are less liable to be affected than children and youths growing up.

This complaint at first puts on the appearance of a common cold, and Dr. Cullen makes mention of instances which never assumed any other shape than that of a cold, although they were obviously the effects of this contagion. But this is not commonly the case. Generally in the course of the second week, or at farthest in the third, the convulsive motion which gives the name to this disease, manifestly shews itself, and is commonly called a *whoop*. This whoop, together with the circumstance of the general spread of the disorder, sufficiently distinguish it.

"The chin cough," says Dr. Darwin, "consists in an inflammation of the membrane which lines the air vessels of the lungs. The whole of the lungs are probably not infected at the same time, but the contagious inflammation continues gradually to creep on the membrane." This opinion seems to account very well for its long continuance, which is from one month to three, and sometimes much longer. "This complaint is not usually classed among febrile disorders, but a fever may generally be perceived to attend it during some part of the day, especially in weak patients. And a general inflammation of the lungs frequently supervenes, and destroys great numbers of children, except the lancet, or four or six leeches be immediately and repeatedly used.

When the child has permanent difficulty of

*breathing which continues between the coughing fits ; unless blood be taken from him, he dies in two, three, or four days, of the inflammation of the lungs.** During this permanent difficulty of breathing the hooping cough abates or quite ceases. Many have been deceived by this circumstance unfortunately supposing the child to be better. But after once or twice bleeding the cough returns, which is then a good symptom, as the child possessing the power to cough is relieved, and once more breathes with ease."

The remedies in this disease are :

1. Gentle vomits of tartar emetic ; this article should be given in small doses frequently repeated till it produces the intended effect.

2. Mild purges repeated so as to keep the bowels gently loose and open.

3. Blisters to be frequently repeated, they may be applied to one or both sides of the breast.

4. Warm bath. This is an excellent remedy where the cough is violent and the child much exhausted. The bath should be a little above blood heat.

5. In every instance where there is diffi-

---

* This is a very important point, and should be particularly observed.

culty of breathing between the fits of coughing, the only safe remedy is copious bleeding. If this be neglected or omitted, the child may die.

6. Young children should lie with their heads and shoulders raised, and should be constantly watched day and night to prevent them from strangling in the cough. A little bow of whale bone or of elastic wood should be used to extract the phlegm out of the mouths of infants. The application of a handkerchief to their mouths when in the act of coughing might suffocate them.

7. After the disease has continued some weeks, and especially if the patient be much reduced, the following dose calculated for a child three or four years old may be useful. Say, calomel one sixth part of a grain, opium one sixth of a grain, rhubarb two grains, to be combined and repeated twice a day. But opium will be very pernicious as long as blood-letting is proper.

8. Towards the close of the complaint all feeble patients should be daily carried out on horseback. This is a most excellent remedy.

CHAPTER XXIX.

MEASLES.

This disease is epidemic. It depends on a specific contagion, and occurs most frequently in children. No age however is exempted from it if the person have not been subjected to it before. It commonly first appears in the month of January, and ceases after the middle of summer; but by various accidents it may be produced at other times of the year.

The symptoms as given by Dr. Cullen are nearly as follows. " The disease always begins with a cold chill which is soon followed by the usual symptoms of fever; as thirst, heat, loss of appetite, anxiety, sickness and vomiting; and these are more or less considerable in different cases. In many instances the fever for the first two days is inconsiderable; but sometimes it is violent from the beginning, and always becomes violent before the eruption appears.

This fever is always attended with hoarseness, with a frequent hoarse dry cough, and often with some difficulty of breathing. The eyelids are swelled, the eyes inflamed and watery. There is a discharge from the nose, with frequent sneezing. In most instances the patient is drowsy in the beginning.

The eruption commonly appears upon the fourth day; first on the face, and successively on the lower parts of the body. Is shews itself first in small red points, which collect together in clusters on the face, and where they are easily perceived to be a little elevated by the sense of touch; but they can scarcely be felt on other parts of the body. The redness of the face continues and sometimes increases for two days. On the third day the vivid redness is changed to a brownish red, and in a day or two more, the eruption entirely disappears, and is followed by a branny scale. During the whole time of the eruption the face appears full, but not much swelled.

Sometimes the fever disappears as soon as the eruption takes place, but this is seldom the case; more commonly it continues, or is increased after the eruption, and in some instances even after the branny scales appear. As long as the fever exists in any considerable degree, the cough continues, and that generally with an increase of the difficulty of breathing. Sometimes an inflammation of the lungs takes place. This is a very serious circumstance when it occurs, and ought to be specially observed.

All the above symptoms admit of very great variation, and in some cases there will be in addition to them, soreness of the throat spitting of blood mixed with the phlegm coughed up, gripes, diarrhoea, and bloody stools. *I suppose that fourteen days intervene between the time of receiving the infection and the appearance of the disease.*

It may be well to observe that the eruption does not invariably appear on the third or fourth day, but varies even to the eighth. Neither does the eruption disappear invariably on a certain day, nor in an unchanging manner; nor is it always followed by the branny scales.

The fever attending the measles is in most instances of the inflammatory kind; but by improper management, or neglect, as well as by the predisposing circumstances attending the patient, it may assume a different form. The remedies to be employed in this disorder are,

1. Blood-letting. This is always necessary when there is a full pulse attended with great pain and violent cough; and that too in every stage of the disease, whether before or after the eruption takes place; or even after the eruption has entirely disappeared.

2. Vomits. A dose of ipecacuanha, will generally remove the sickness at the stomach.

3. Soothing drinks, such as barley-water; balm tea; flax-seed tea; cider and water

made very weak; vinegar and water; apple water; dried cherry-water, &c. These moisten the throat and afford much relief.

4. Blisters. After sufficient evacuation, by bleeding or otherwise, blisters may be applied to the neck and sides. They prevent injury to the lungs.

5. Opiates. If the pulse be soft and the patient labour under the distressing symptoms of diarrhoea and cough, opium may be used not only at night, but at any time during the day. This remedy however, will seldom be proper earlier than the fifth or sixth day.

In most instances if the patient be kept cool, and take opening and cooling drinks, &c. If he be bled when the symptoms are violent, as also about the time the measles disappear or when the branny scale presents itself; and if his bowels be opened on the third and fourth day of the eruption, with cream of tartar, flowers of sulphur, manna or the like; little else will be wanting especially in childrens cases.

☞ Here let it be particularly observed, that in every instance where the eruption seems to take place with difficulty, and where the pulse is full and tight with other marks of great fever, all spirituous liquors and other heating medicines are highly pernicious. In such cases sufficient bleeding would be much more proper.

It may be useful also to observe that there is a fever which sometimes takes place during the prevalence of the measles, very much resembling that disease, even assuming the appearance of an eruption. But persons are still liable to take the true measles after having been subjected to this disease. It is sometimes attended with symptoms of the croup, See chap. xxiv. Distinction 2d. In that case the treatment must be the same as if croup were the original disorder; in all other respects the remedies useful in measles might be employed in this kind of fever.

Patients when recovering from the measles are frequently subject to diarrhoea. This uncomfortable symptom may be removed by moderate doses of opium frequently repeated. The drinks recommended above, article 3d will also be of use.

Sore eyes sometimes follow the measles. These are to be cured by blistering the temples, and back of the neck, and washing the eyes with a weak solution of white vitriol.

A cough and fever frequently attend for some time after the eruption disappears. These are to be relieved by a vegetable diet, warmth, and gently riding out in the fresh and open air.

☞ When the measles are expected, it will be found beneficial to prepare for them, by living chiefly on milk and vegetable diet, and by avoiding every kind of spirituous liquors.

CHAPTER XXX.

PUTRID SORE-THROAT.

This is a fever from contagion. It generally appears in autumn, from September to December. Children and women are more subject to it than men, and persons with black eyes are more subject to its attacks than others. More boys recover from it than girls. It generally follows moist, wet and hazy weather.

The principal symptoms attending it are great weakness; slight eruption; weak and quick pulse; ulcers in the throat; delirium especially at night; diarrhoea; inflamed and watery eyes; and a flat and ratling voice. The ulcers and sloughs in the throat are of a whitish ash color, and the breath of the patient is very offensive to the smell. The remedies are,

1. Blood-letting for the first three days.

2. Pukes. Say ipecac. ten grains and calomel four grains, to be taken together as a dose for a child of eight or ten years old.

3. Bark, wine and cordial aliment. The bark should be given in substance.* But if that be impracticable, a decoction may be substituted. Port wine should be prefered. If wine cannot be had, a decoction of *Virginia Snakeroot;* (commonly called *black snakeroot*) is a tolerable substitute. Chicken broth is the best diet, and should be used as early as possible in the disease.

4. Blisters should be applied to the neck and throat. But blisters drawn in this disease should never be dressed with colewart leaves; some kind of mild ointment spread on a bit of fine linen should be prefered. For this purpose melt together oil five parts, and bees-wax one part.

5. The mouth and throat should be washed with barley water or very thin gruel, to which should be added a little vinegar and honey, and if convenient a portion of the tincture of myrrh. Sixty or eighty drops of the tincture of myrrh might be added to half an ounce of the gruel, &c. or if the myrrh cannot be had, as much calomel as

* The bark waistcoat may be worn throughout the whole course of the disease, and for some time afterwards, even till fully recovered.

may be sufficient to turn it of a whitish color, will be a good substitute.

☞ I have found great benefit from frequently washing the mouth and throat well with the following mixture. Take salt petre half an ounce and borax one quarter of an ounce; the whole to be dissolved in one pint of water and sweetened with honey. I have used it successfully in a number of cases without any other topical application.

6. The steams of vinegar and myrrh received into the throat by the help of a funnel are sometimes beneficial. The following will often answer a very good purpose after blood-letting:

7. Wash the throat with a decoction of equal parts of the bark of persimmon tree, sumac root, and briar root. Let it be made pretty strong, and add to one quart, as much alum as is equal in bulk to a middle sized chesnut.

8. Touch the ulcers twice a day, with a soft moss dipped in a tincture of equal parts of burnt alum and blue stone, (blue vitriol) dissolved in rum or brandy. Put in as much as will dissolve.

CHAPTER XXXI.

SCARLET FEVER.

This fever like the foregoing, depends on a specific contagion. It comes on with chilliness, sickness at the stomach and vomiting. These symptoms are specially characteristic of the disease. There are in some cases a swelling of the throat, and difficulty of speaking, swallowing and breathing. Sometimes there is a squeaking voice and ulcers in the throat, which are in some instances deep and covered with white, brown or black sloughs. A thick mucus is discharged from the nose, sometimes from the beginning, but more commonly coming on about the fifth day. An eruption appears on the skin, sometimes preceding, sometimes following the swelling and ulcers of the throat. In some, the eruption is confined to the outside of the throat and breast; in others wholly to the limbs. In some, it appears on the second and third day, and never afterwards. In some, it appears with the sore throat, and perhaps in others without it. The bowels are generally regular but some have diarrhoea.

This fever is moderately inflammatory and differs from the malignant or putrid sore throat in the following particulars.

1. It is not always attended with a sore throat.

2. The eruption in this fever is of a deeper red color, and is more smooth, resembling the back of a boiled lobster.

3. The skin is also more hot and dry.

4. The skin peals off in the close of this fever.

5. It is not so dangerous as the putrid sore throat.

6. It commonly goes off with a swelling of the hands and feet.

7. And lastly it frequently appears in summer and dry weather.

Again this fever may be distinguished from a common inflammation of the almonds, &c. called quinsey, by the following remarks.

1. The appearance of ulcers in common quinsey, is confined to the almonds, &c.

2. A strong full and tense pulse attend an inflammatory quinsey, always admitting the use of the lancet.

3. A common quinsey is not attended with external redness.

The remedies for the scarlet fever are,

1. Puking. Ipecacuanha and calomel combined as in the foregoing disease, chap. xxix. This preparation is to be prefered before all others, it is a certain cure if given on or before

the first day. The dose should be repeated according to the violence of the disease.

2. Small doses of calomel. If the patient should be very weak small doses of opium should be added to the calomel, to prevent its purgative effects.

3. Blisters should be applied behind the ears and on the throat.

4. The throat to be washed as in chap. xxx. except that in the first stages of this disease, the best gargle perhaps is a solution of salt petre with the addition of borax, but it must not be quite so strong as advised for the putrid sore throat. Calomel is a proper article to be applied to the ulcers in the throat, see article 4th, under the head of putrid sore throat.

5. Snuff may be used about the fifth day to excite a running at the nose.

6. Towards the close of the disease, wine and water or wine whey may be used to such extent only as to keep up a very gentle perspiration.

7. Whenever the swelling of the extremities takes place, a few doses of calomel may be repeated.

It is worthy of observation, that this disease can be communicated before it can be known to be present in any case. It is therefore unnecessary to remove children out of the family where it makes its appearance.

Some are of opinion that the scarlet fever might be prevented by using occasional doses of rhubarb. This remedy is worthy of a trial.

CHAPTER XXXII.

INFLAMMATION OF THE EYES.

Sore eyes are of two kinds.

1. That which effects the coats of the ball of the eye, &c.

2. That which affects the eye-lids only.

The causes inducing inflammation are,

1. External violence, wounds, particles of dust, sand, &c. or the hairs of the eye-lids inverted.

2. Too much light or strong light too long continued, sitting up at night before a fire, riding in snow, particularly when it falls early or late in the season, writing or reading too much at night, and too long accurately inspecting very minute objects.

3. Frequent intoxication.

4. Sharp matter, such as tobacco, &c. received into the eye.

5. Sympathy. Sore eyes are frequently taken by looking at others in that condition, and is the effect of an active imagination.

6. General fever sometimes induces this disease.

The remedies are as follows :

1. Bleeding. When there is general fever, copious bleeding from the arm will be necessary. If no general fever be present, cupping the temples and scarifying the inside of the eye-lids.

2. Purges. These may be more or less violent according to the violence of the disease.

3. Blisters. These should be applied to the neck, behind the ears, and to the temples.

4. Certain washes. These must be mild or sharp according to the stage of the disease. In most instances when an inflammation of the eyes first appear, cold water, milk and water or mild lead water will be proper. The lead water should be made into a poultice and applied to the eye affected, first covering it with a bit of cambric or muslin.

5. In the last stages of this disease the eyes may be washed with the following solution, white vitriol and sugar of lead of each forty grains, spring water one gill. If this be not convenient, weak spirit and wa-

ter,* Madeira wine and water, salt and water or a decoction of oak bark and leaves not too strong.

In curing this disease, the patient should not be exposed to the light; and all spirituous liquors must be carefully avoided.

When they are particles of dust or the like in the eye, it may sometimes be washed out with clean water. If an inverted hair be the cause, it must be plucked out.

If the disease should be of long standing and be obstinate, setons and issues will be proper.

CHAPTER XXXIII

BURNS.

If fever be excited by a burn the patient should be bled, and purged with gentle laxative medicines. But the greatest dependance should be placed upon applications to be made to the part affected. Tar, lead water, rum and water, holding the part affected near to the fire, or in cold water; the part should be immersed and kept covered with the water, for one or more hours. Oil is an

* Say water five spoonsful, brandy or rum one spoonful.

improper application. A strong solution of soap and water is a good application. An ointment made of James-town weed, (*stramonium*) is said to be an excellent remedy, after the inflammation is subdued. Cold and salted dough made of Indian corn meal is a good application, especially where the skin is unbroken.

Spirit of turpentine diluted with rum or brandy of such strength as just to be tolerably well borne, is the best and safest application to a burn. This or tar ought always to be applied where the injury done by the fire is considerable.

CHAPTER XXXIV.

BLEEDING AT THE NOSE.

I. This may be the effect of too strong a circulation of the blood towards the head, and in that case the patient should,

1. Let blood as often as may be necessary.

2. Cold application should be made to his head, and should frequently be repeated. I have known the application of a cloth wetted with cold water made to the groin, to afford instant relief.

II. Debility sometimes may be the predisposing cause. When this is the case, laudnum, blisters, and common salt are the proper remedies.

The preventative remedies are gentle exercise with a milk and vegetable diet.

CHAPTER XXXV.

SCALD HEAD AND TETTERS.

For the cure of scald head and tetter worms, the first thing necessary is to cleanse the part affected, by carefully washing it with milk and water.

2. Apply mild poultices, changing them every four hours for two or three days.—Then apply a solution of ten grains of corosive sublimate dissolved in one pint of spring water. Some recommend a tar ointment, others a stiff plaister of pitch so as ultimately to extirpate the hairs, as the best remedies for scalded head. Others recommend a decoction of tobacco; strong solution of soap and water, &c. &c.

CHAPTER XXXVI.

WHITE SWELLING OF THE JOINTS.

On the first attack of this disease, "apply eight or more leeches and afterwards small blisters to the joint; gentle frictions of the part; two or three vomits a week, with entire rest of the limb; and in the end sea-bathing," or a bath of salt and water.

Electricity ought to be used in every case where it can be done. This remedy will frequently succeed when the appearances are unfavourable.

Early application should be made to an able physician. Too often by an unaccountable kind of neglect the lives of very promising children are lost.

CHAPTER XXXVII.

MUMPS.

This disease is often epidemic, and manifestly contagious. It comes on with the usual symptoms of fever, and is soon after attended with a considerable swelling of the throat and neck. The swelling at first seems to be fixed in a moveable lump at the corner of the lower jaw, but it soon spreads itself over a great part of the neck. Sometimes it is confined to one side of the neck, but more commonly both sides are affected.

The swelling continues to increase till the fourth day. From that time it declines, and in a few days more passes off entirely.

As the swelling of the throat goes off, it affects the testicles in the male sex, or the breasts in the female.

The fever attending this disease is commonly slight and goes off with the swelling of the neck. Sometimes however, when the swelling of the testicles does not succeed to that of the neck, or when one or the other has been suddenly checked by cold or otherwise, the fever becomes very considerable. Fever under these circumstances is sometimes attended with delirium, and has in some cases proved fatal.

As this disease commonly runs its course, without either dangerous or troublesome symptoms, so it seldom requires any remedies.

A cooling regimen, and care to avoid cold, are all that will be commonly necessary.

But when upon the disappearance of the swelling of the testicles in males, or of the breasts in females, the fever becomes considerable,

Then

1. Let blood according to circumstances and repeat it daily till the fever abates.

2. Give one or more gentle purges. Even calomel and jalap would not be amiss.

3. Warm steam should be applied to the breast or testicle. It is a very convenient method to take a newly opened gourd of suitable size. Put into it a few mullen leaves—Scald the inside of the gourd and its contents—Pour off the water, and let the testicles or breasts, as the case may be, hang down into the gourd. Continue to repeat the application three or four times a day so long as it is necessary. At each application the part affected should be made to sweat freely.

This mode of sweating is useful whenever either the breast or testicle is affected with painful swelling from whatever cause.

CHAPTER XXXVIII.

COMMON QUINSEY.

This disease is an inflammation of the soft membrance of the inside of the throat. It chiefly affects those parts commonly called the almonds; but frequently spreads itself so as to affect every part of the throat.

It first shews itself by some swelling and redness of the parts. As the parts swell it becomes more painful and difficult to swallow—the pain sometimes shooting into the ear. There will be a troublesome clamminess of the mouth and throat, with a frequent but difficult discharge of phlegm. And there is commonly considerable fever.

This disease is never contagious. It is commonly occasioned by cold externally applied, particularly about the neck. Young and robust people are most liable to it's attack. Persons once affected with it are therefore the more easily affected a second time. It occurs most commonly in spring and autumn, when there are the most frequent changes of weather.

For the cure of this disease,

1. Bleed, as far as the general fever may make it necessary—Leeches applied to the throat and blistering the same, may be found useful in some cases.

2. A full dose of tartar emetic given as a puke, must be useful in a great majority of instances.

3. Warm steam frequently inhaled into the throat by the help of the spout of a teapot, or funnel, or other instrument. For

this purpose hot water, to which is added a little vinegar, may be used.

4. Gargles. Sage tea and honey. A decoction of roses and honey. A decoction such as is recommended under the article of *putrid sore throat*. Any of these may be used at discretion.

5. Frequent purges repeated from the first to the fifth day if necessary. Glaubers salts answers this intention very well.

6. Sweating medicines are generally useful., After one or two bleedings and purgings—take, tartar emet. three grains, spring water two gills, laudanum three tea spoonsfull—of this preparation one table spoonfull may be given every second or third hour.

7. If the swelling progress obstinately, notwithstanding all these remedies—then repeat the use of warm steam till the tumor breaks ; or if it should not break of itself, it should be opened with a lancet or other proper instrument.

Note. When it is reduced to a certainty, that the quinsey cannot be scattered, warm poultices may be applied externally.

CHAPTER XXXIX.

CATARRH, COMMONLY CALLED A BAD COLD.

This disease commonly begins with some difficulty of breathing through the nose, and with a sense of fullness stopping up that passage. There is commonly some dull pain and a sense of weight felt in the forehead, as also some stiffness and soreness in the motion of the eyes.

After a short time, a thin watery and hot fluid flows from the eyes and nose, more particularly from the latter; and this fluid sometimes is so acrid as to excoriate the cuticle, or outer coat of the skin, over which it passes.

There is also pretty commonly a peculiar kind of indolence and weakness felt over the whole body. Some cold shiverings are felt, or at least the patient is more than ordinarily sensible to the coldness of the air.

The pulse becomes frequent, especially towards evening.

Before many days a troublesome cough—a hoarseness—a sense of roughness and soreness in the air pipes—and a difficulty of breathing take place.

The cough is at first dry, occasioning pains about the chest, and more especially in the breast. Sometimes pains resembling rheu matism are felt in several parts of the body, particularly about the head and neck. There will however be a considerable increase of thirst.

In young people the case remains but a few days in the above condition before the cough becomes more effectual, and the phlegm coughed up is ticker and more white. The mucus from the nose is also thicker and less corroding to the skin. The appetite returns, and the patient gradually recovers ordinary health.

But when the violence of the disease is considerable, or when there is danger of consumption from heriditary predisposition, it is certainly most safe, and often it is absolutely necessary, to have recourse to suitable remedies.

For the cure,

1. Where there is considerable fever the patient should be bled—And this remedy should be daily repeated as often as the violence of the symptoms make it necessary.

2. A full dose of tartar emetic or ipecacuanha.

3. The patient should live on a light diet, abstain from all laborious exercise, and in violent cases even from walking about the

house, and there should be no fresh application of cold.

4. Gentle purges frequently repeated will much assist the cure.

5. Warm diluting drinks should be freely taken, especially at night—such as flax-seed tea, mallows tea, or even weak hyson tea. If one tenth or one twentieth part of a grain of tartar emetic were added to a free drink, at intervals of two or three hours, it would be the more effectual.

6. Occasional doses of salt petre from five to ten grains at a time, well diluted in one of the above drinks.

7. After five or six days blisters may be repeated according to existing circumstances.

8. Heat applied to the skin before going to bed at night. After proper evacuation the patient may sit or stand near a good fire, turning side for side until very warm. This will be found a good general stimulant.

9. After the fever and pains subside, the patient should gradually return to his usual habits.

It may not be improper to observe here, that, an affection like the common catarrh, or *bad cold*, sometimes spreads itself in a speedy manner over a very extensive tract of country ; nay sometimes not even confining itself to one continent. This complaint is commonly called an *Influenza*, and in its progress attacks old and young almost without distinction.

In this affection the treatment proper in common cold is likewise proper.

For the use of those who have no better source of information, I will also add the following observations.

When a violent catarrh or influenza seizes upon old people, particularly those of a fleshy habit of body, or those who have been in habits of drinking ardent spirits freely, it is very apt to affect their lungs with bastard pleurisy, *(peripneumonia notha.)* In such cases large blood-letting would certainly be very pernicious. Rather treat them as follows, viz.

1. Let them be kept warm and take freely warm diluting drinks.

2. One or more doses of ipecacuanha or tartar emetic, may be necessary.

3. The violence of the fever should be moderated by using gentle laxative medicines.

4. Blisters may be freely used.

5. After a few days hore-hound tea may be taken pretty largely.

6. Warm steam may be frequently inhaled into the lungs—especially if the cough becomes dry.

7. If sweating can be procured by using warm teas only, it is very well; but no strong medicine should be given for that purpose till after the fifth or sixth day, when small doses of the rattle-snake root might be used with advantage.

8. Warmth, and composure of mind are indispensable.

9. Elixir paregoric is a valuable remedy in the last stages of this complaint, in the cases now under consideration. Thirty to sixty drops the dose, to be repeated every eighth hour.

Note. Blood-letting may be necessary in some cases, but it should be done under the direction of much experience and judgment only.

CHAPTER XL.

SOME REMARKS ON THE MEDICINES PRESCRIBED IN THE COURSE OF THIS WORK.

1. *Allum*, is used in floodings and in long continued fluxes. It is given to grown persons in doses of five to twenty grains every four, eight, or twelve hours, according to the exigency of the case. In women's cases it may commonly be mixed with kino, which see.

2. *Aloes Succoterine*, is a purgative medicine, very stimulating to the rectum or lower intestine, and if too frequently used, induces *piles*. It is however a very good article in cases of *suppressed menses*, *worms*, *&c.* The dose for grown persons may be from six to sixty grains. For a child of two years old, from two to six grains.

3. *Assa Foetida*, is used in hysteric cases. In hysteric suffocation, a plaister made of assafoetida one quarter of an ounce, and camphor ten to fifteen grains, may be applied to the stomach, and will be found a useful remedy.

4. *Bark*. Of this article there are two kinds, viz. the *red* and *pale*. It is a useful remedy in feeble habits, and strengthens the stomach and bowels. It is employed in the cure of fever and ague ; but it is sometimes unsuccessful unless the patient be first bled one or more times. Its dose for a man may be from thirty to sixty grains, to be repeated every one, two or three hours. A dose for a child of two years old, from five to ten grains.

5. *Borax*, is used to relieve children in thrush, it is also proper for making gargarisms in cases of sore throat, whether in scarlet fever or putrid sore throat. In cases of thrush it may be prepared as follows : Take

borax sixty grains, honey one ounce, and it is better to add as much water as may serve to dilute it sufficiently. It is said to be useful as a medicine to be taken inwardly in cases of fluor albus. The dose from five grains to sixty. If taken in this disease, a few grains of nutmeg or cinnamon should be added to each dose, otherwise it may produce vomiting.

6. *Calomel*, is an excellent medicine. It may be used as a purge either alone or combined with jalap. If it be intended to operate speedily, it should be combined. If not it is most effectual by itself. Sometimes when given too often, or in too large doses, it produces a salivation. The dose for a man is from five to twenty grains, for a child of two years old from two to four grains ; if given for worms it might be combined with a little aloes or jalap. In all billious fevers it is a very useful remedy, and after sufficient evacuation by bleeding, &c. it may be given in small doses, frequently repeated, with very great advantage.

7. *Camphor*, is a very powerful stimulant and is sometimes useful in fever after sufficient depletion. It produces sweating and may be given in doses from two to twenty grains. It is sometimes useful, combined with salt petre. When dissolved in spirit, it

is sometimes useful as an external application for the relief of pain, inflammation, numbness, palsey, &c.

8. *Carolina Pink Root.** Perhaps the dose of this article as advised in chap. XXII. part IV. may be too strong. It will be safest to make trial as follows. Take one quarter of an ounce, stew it gently in one pint of water down to three gills. Give half a gill of this decoction to a child six years old, morning and evening, and observe its effects. If it procures unusual drowsiness, the dose may be considered too strong, and ought therefore to be lessened or entirely omitted.

9. *Castor Oil*, is a mild and pleasant purge ; its dose for a man is from one to two table-spoonsfull, for a child of two or three years old from one to two tea-spoonsfull.†

10. *Camomile Flowers*, make a tea which is useful in weakly cases, as of indigestion, sickness at the stomach from weakness, &c.

11. *Columbo*, is said to be a most a specific in cholera morbus, nausea, vomiting, purging, diarrhoea, dissentery, billious fevers, indigestion, want of appetite, and most dis-

---

* Add to each portion of pink-root a sufficient quantity of senna to make it act gently as a purge.

† Frequent doses of castor-oil during the last two months of pregnancy will certainly conduce to an easy and safe delivery.

orders of the stomach and bowels where no inflammation exists. But on the principles of Dr. Rush's theory, in every species of cholic, blood letting ought to be the first remedy, and afterwards perhaps gentle evacuants. Then if debility prevail, the columbo with orange peel, &c. would be proper. From ten to thirty grains every three or four hours the common dose; but it may be extended even to one sixth of an ounce.

12. *Cream of Tartar*, is a very mild purge, and may be given from one to two ounces. If dissolved in a large quantity of warm water, and taken in a gradual manner, it evacuates the intestines in a mild and effectual way. Combined with jalap, it is considerably effectual in exciting the action of the absorbents; by these means I once cured an ascites, that is a dropsy of the belly, of long standing.

13. *Cinnamon*. An excellent aromatic, and considerably strengthening to the bowels, and is recommended in cases of flooding, whites, &c.

14. *Ether*, if applied externally relieves pains, and if given internally it removes flatulency, asthma, hiccup, &c. If applied to an inflammation and is suffered to evaporate, it will cool and relieve it wonderfully. If applied to chronic rheumatism in a state of con-

liniment so as to prevent its evaporation, as with a cloth wetted with it and covered with the palm of the hand, it will relieve the pain on opposite principles.

15. *Elixir Vitriol*, is a valuable remedy in weakness of the stomach, indigestion, &c. but being considerably stimulant, it must be improper when the pulse is tense, and in all cases of inflammation. Its dose from ten to thirty drops, in a cup of some kind of liquid. If this article be dropped on linnen or cotton cloaths, it destroys them.

16. *Flies*, called also *Cantharides*, are used for the purpose of drawing blisters. Perhaps the best mode of applying them is in the form of a quilt. If prepared in this form, one quilt will serve three or four times, when applied on plaisters, the skin should be guarded by applying a thin bit of muslin between it and the flesh. The application of cantharides sometimes excites a strangury. See chap. XV. part II. When this circumstance takes place, the patient should drink plentifully of some diluting draught. A tea made of mullen would answer a good purpose in this case. He should also take a dose of opium, and repeat it in eight hours if necessary. Blisters are seldom proper till the violence of a fever is reduced by bleeding and purging. They should not be dressed

with colewort leaves. Some kind of mild ointment should be preferred.

17. *Ipecacuanha* is an excellent puke, and is the mildest and safest of any yet known. Its dose for grown persons is from five to thirty grains, and for a child of two years old from one to five grains. It may be taken in a cup of tea or in the form of bolus, and while it operates the patient may drink freely of weak camomile tea.

18. *Iron* is one of the most powerful strengtheners. In weak lax, and pale habits, such as cachexy, green sickness, it is the best medicine as yet known. But it is often injudiciously employed so as to do irreparable damage. If there be tension, rigidity and spasmodic stricture existing in the system, it is highly pernicious. Let it therefore be observed that if the use of this article excite pain in the head, with other feverish symptoms, it should not be continued. It may be given in the form of simple filings, rust of iron, or the salt of steel. If the rust or filings be used, the dose may be from five to ten grains; if salt of steel be chosen, from one to three grains may be the dose. It is generally the best method to administer it in small doses, frequently repeated. Cases may occur in which this article is really necessary and in which, notwithstanding its

propriety, it may cause considerable sickness and pertubations. In such instances a moderate dose of opium may be given after each dose, or the patient may be directed to take it on going to bed at night, and again half an hour before rising up in the morning ; and at other times of the day let him or her walk moderately immediately after taking the dose.

19. *Jalap* is an excellent purge, if it be ground together with cream of tartar it will operate in smaller doses than when taken singly ; and it will furthermore act more gently and without griping. Ground together with hard sugar, it becomes a good and safe medicine for children. Combined with calomel, it is a most powerful purge. Its dose for a man is from twenty to forty grains, for a child two or three years old, f[illegible]n five to eight or ten grains. In cases of billious fever, after bleeding, when that evacuation is required, ten grains of jalap with five grains of calomel might be taken every three or four hours 'till a sufficient effect is produced.

20. *Kino* is an astringent gum and is useful in diseases of laxity, such as diarrhoea, fluor albus, &c, it may be given in the following form. Take kino two parts and allum three parts, grind them together ; of this mixture

the dose may be from five to fifteen grains, every three or four hours. In cases where the allum is improper or disagreeable, from five to fifteen grains of the kino alone, it may be dissolved in water or a solution of gum arabic, to which may also be added a few drops of laudanum.

21. *Magnesia* is a very mild article, it corrects acidity in the stomach and in the first passages. Hence its effects in relieving heart burn, as also giddiness, vomiting, and pain in the stomach, when they are the consequences of an acid matter collected in the stomach. It also relieves gripes in children when brought on by the same cause. Its dose for an infant may be from two to five grains, to be given in a tea of fennel seed, and repeated. The addition of a small portion of rhubarb or manna gives it a little more activity as a purge.

22. *Manna* is one of the mildest purgatives, and may be given with great safety to children and pregnant women. It is proper in pleurisy, all inflammatory fevers, and such other cases as may require mild purges. Its dose is from half an ounce to two ounces; and it is best perhaps to dissolve it in a decoction of cassia, which is an inferior kind of cinnamon. If a little tartar emetic or some other active article be added, the manna will

operate much more effectually. Say manna half an ounce, tartar emetic half a grain, to be repeated every two or three hours. *This would be an excellent preparation as a purge in child-bed fever.*

23. *Gum Myrrh* is a stimulating medicine and is admissible in those cases only where iron is proper, as in chlorosis, &c. Its dose may be from five grains to thirty; a tincture may be made of this gum as follows: Take gum myrrh three ounces, proof spirit or good wine, one pint and a half, digest them ten days with a gentle heat. The tincture so prepared is a useful addition to cleansing gargarisms, such as are proper in putrid sore throat, &c.

24. *Nutmeg* is warm and agreeable to the taste, is good for the stomach, corrects a laxative habit, relieves indigestion, &c. its dose is from six grains to thirty, if roasted in substance, it is said to be more astringent and is an excellent remedy in chronic diarrhoes and dissenteries.

25. *Orange-peel* is employed as a stomachic medicine, it promotes appetite, gives strength and vigor to the bowels, and is therefore proper in cases of indigestion, flatulency when the consequence of debility, &c. It is rendered more effectual by joining it with columbo, the yellow outside rind should be

preferred; infusions with water are better than any preparation with ardent spirit. In all cases where bitters are required, the use of spirit must be injurious. Wine, if good, might be useful.

26. *Olive Oil*, called also *Sweet Oil*, is employed as an external application, it is improper however in cases of burns, especially if the skin peel off. But I intend in a particular manner to recommend a frequent use of it internally, to such women as are wont to have hard labours. They should begin its use several days before the time of delivery. One or two ounces should be beaten up with one or more yolks of eggs till it will readily mix with water, then add half a pint or a pint of water sweetened with manna or syrrup. With this she should keep her bowels constantly lax. Where there is sufficient strength, blood letting should also be employed.

27. *Opium* is a powerful cordial, it eases pain, but at the same time very much increases the circulation, and is therefore very injurious in inflammatory fevers, especially if the brain, lungs, liver, stomach or bowels, &c. be the seat of the disease, at least considerable evacuations should be procured before it is ever employed in such cases. It is never proper if there be tensity in the pulse.

In cases of external tumor and consequent pain, it is frequently admissible, and when debility prevails with a soft and languid pulse, it is an excellent remedy. Its dose when taken in substance may be from one to three grains, in a liquid form, as laudanum or tincture of opium, which are two different names for the same thing, the dose may be from twenty-five to sixty drops. But it should be remembered that this article generally induces costiveness.

28. *Precipitate of Mercury* is either *red* or *white*. If applied in dry powder to a foul ulcer, they cleanse it. When combined with mild ointment or hogs-lard, they form a drying ointment, useful in eruptions on the skin, sore nipples, &c. Take lard, or rather sweet oil hardened sufficiently by melting bees-wax together with it, half an ounce; precipitate forty to sixty grains, mix them in a cold state, and the ointment is prepared.

29. *Rhubarb* is a mild purge, and may be given in doses from twenty to sixty grains, but as it is considerably astringent, it should not be employed where a costive habit is to be avoided. In chronic diarrhoeas, it may be given in small doses of five or six grains, combined with opium, two or three times a day. It cannot be a proper remedy in inflammatory cases, and is therefore forbidden in

dyssentery ; but in cases of debility, it is frequently useful ; combined with manna it will evacuate the intestines without exhausting the strength of the patient in any considerable degree.

30. *Russian Castor* is useful in hysteric cases, see part I. chap. XXIII. But it may also be used in form of a tincture. Take castor one ounce, proof spirit two pounds, digest ten days, and it is ready for use ; the dose may be from twenty to sixty drops. It is sometimes taken to advantage in conjunction with laudanum, say laudanum twenty-five drops, tincture of castor twenty-five drops, the whole for one dose in hysteric suffocation, as also in painful menstruation where blood letting is not needed.

31. *Sal Ammoniac*, of this one ounce may be dissolved in one quart of water or of spirit and water combined. This solution is useful as an external application in cases of inflamed breasts, &c.

32. *Spirits of Nitre* or *Nitric Ether*, is used in fever, and is an excellent medicine for quenching thirst, expelling flatulences, preventing nausea and vomiting, and moderately strengthening the stomach ; it is diaphoretic and cooling. The dose may vary from twenty to forty drops.

33. *Spirits of Sal Ammoniac* and *Spirits of Hartshorn* are similar in their nature and effects, but the first is perhaps the best. The dose may be from fifteen drops to sixty ; it is useful in faintings and other hysteric affections ; if given in wine whey it generally procures a very pleasant sweat.

34. *Salt Petre*, called also *Nitre*, is a useful remedy in inflammatory fever. The dose may vary from three grains to forty, every two hours. It is most effectual if given immediately after its solution. Some caution however is necessary in using this article, as it sometimes occasions a nausea or pain in the stomach. In such cases it requires plentiful dilution, and sometimes the addition of a little camphor. Nitre is an excellent ingredient in gargarisms and mouth waters.

35. *Salt of Tartar*, called also *Fixed Alkali*, is used for making the saline mixture. Take salt of tartar twenty grains, lime juice or vinegar as much as may saturate it, or till it ceases to effervesce ; pure water one and a half ounces, and syrrup two ounces. The whole may be taken in the course of four hours, to be repeated as often as may be thought necessary. It may be given also in a simple solution, with pure water ; in this shape the dose may be from ten to thirty or more grains. But it should always be suffi-

ciently diluted. Every three or four grains require one ounce of water. The *saline mixture* given in a state of effervescence frequently corrects vomiting. The simple solution of tartar relieves heart burn, &c.

35. *Senna* is a purge of considerable activity, and is commonly taken in form of an infusion. Pour one pint of boiling water on one quarter of an ounce of senna, let it stand several hours in a moderate degree of heat. One gill may be taken every two hours as a dose for a grown person ; and one or two spoonsful for a child two years old. It is rendered more pleasant and mild in its operation, if one ounce of manna be added.—The addition of a small portion of ginger will help to prevent its griping.

37. *Flowers of Sulphur* is a gentle and pleasant purge. It is also effectual in curing affections of the skin, as the itch, &c. combined with the cream of tartar, is useful in piles. It is also a very good purge to be employed on the third and fourth day of the measles.

38. *Tartar Emetic*, called also *Tartarized Antimony*, may be so varied in its dose as to produce sweating, puking, or purging. It is a medicine both safe and convenient, and has but little taste. The dose as a puke is from one grain to five, and may be dissolved in

warm water. When used in children's cases one grain may be dissolved in one ounce of water, which may be sweetened with sugar; a teaspoonful or two may be given every half hour till the patient vomits, if that be the intention. When given to procure sweating, the dose may vary from one eighth to one half of a grain. It may be repeated every two or three hours; and in inflammatory fevers, ten or more grains of nitre should be added to each dose. This is an excellent remedy to be employed in inflammatory cases after sufficient blood-letting. If it be given in small doses, well diluted every half hour, it will act as a purge and the more certainly so, if some mild purgative be added, as manna, purging salts, &c. This last is an excellent remedy in the beginning of fever; and if sufficiently employed, frequently will remove the disease. As the tartar is nearly without taste, it is very easily imposed on obstinate children, by mixing it with cold water and giving it when they ask for drink.

CHAPTER XLI.

A NOTE ON FEVER.

THE NATURE OF FEVER IS BRIEFLY STATED, AND SOME DIRECTIONS ARE GIVEN FOR THE CURE.

A man in habits of labor, will rise early in the morning, and commence his business: he will toil all day, and barely be sensible of fatigue at night.

This ability to continue his labors very much depends on the degree of regularity with which he proceeds. For if he perform more than his usual portion of work, his strength will fail in a much shorter time.

The energies which constitute his strength, and his ability to continue his labors for any longer or shorter duration, depend, first on the state and probably on the operations of the brain; and secondly, on exercise and habit. However much a man may be accustomed to labor, if he be unwell, his strength fails him. However vigorous his health without habitual labor, he will soon be overcome by fatigue. However much fatigued, rest restores his strength. And the more accustomed to labour, the less rest will be sufficient to maintain his strength.

The energies upon which bodily motion, as in labor, running, walking, or the like, depends, are generated in the system, perhaps in the brain and nerves, and are deposited in the muscles. The muscles thus furnished with a capability of motion, are by exercise and habit brought under the influence or command of the will.* But whenever there is a deficiency of such energy, in the proportion of such deficiency the will ceases to maintain its influence or command. *A man very much weakened by fever has very little strength.*

The heart and arteries are endued with a similar energy; that is, with a capability of being put into motion. But these are not under the command of the will, neither can the will have much influence in increasing or lessening their motion.

By physiciaus this energy or capability of motion in the heart and arteries, is called *excitability*.

The motion of the heart and arteries is roused and maintained by other remote powers, which act upon their *excitability*. Such are the *blood itself*, *the nourishment* daily taken in, *the excrements*, *the passions*, *the ef-*

---

* These energies when under the command of the will, are called *strength*.

forts of mind, the noise and bustle of business, bodily labour or exercise, *warmth* &c.

Any of these or other powers, which are naturally, habitually, or accidentally applied to any part or parts of the system, and which on application are capable of producing an increase of motion in the heart and arteries, are called *stimulants*.

The motion thus produced is called *excitement*.

The excitement of the heart and arteries must be continual, for the continual preservation of life; *of course there must be a continual production of excitability*.

The excitability of the blood-vessels, and the voluntary power of the muscles, must be the same principle differently employed. For if there be an extraordinary increase of excitement for any considerable length of time, it will be found, that, there will be a proportionate dimunition of voluntary strength. *Fever always weakens the patient*.

Then of course voluntary muscular motion, as also the excitement of the blood-vessels, must invariably expend a quantity of excitability commensurate to itself. That is, in any given time, say for one day by way of example; then, as in the case of voluntary motion, the more violently a man labors in the morning, the less he will be able to labor in the evening—and the contrary: so also the more violent the excitement in the morning, the same stimulants being applied, the less will be the excitement in the evening—and the contrary. And again, as the man who labors regularly according to his ordinary custom, can continue to labor with uniform strength through the day, so ordinary excitement may likewise be uniform throughout the day.

Consequently if the *quantity of excitement* of the whole mass of blood vessels be exactly proportioned to the *quantity of excitability* constantly generated or furnished, then the excitement will be equable, or natural, or healthful.

If there be an application of more than ordinary stimulants, and if such application be suddenly made, then there will be an increase of excitement; and if the increase be sufficient to induce a sense of languor, and general distress, it is FEVER *directly* produced.*

If the quantity of stimulants acting upon the blood vessels, be less than natural, the quantity of excitement will also be less than natural, and of course there will be an *accu-*

* Fever in this state may be almost universally cured by bleeding and purging only. Sometimes by puking and purging only; and sometimes by either one of the three remedies.

mulation of excitability. For excitability is considered to be uniformly generated, if the energies of the brain remain the same.

If such increase of excitability become considerable, it must therefore follow that the ordinary quantity of stimulants, or even less than the ordinary quantity, would be capable of producing an increase of excitement. *This is fever indirectly produced.*

It would seem that excitability can be generated and conveyed to the muscles or blood-vessels, whilst they themselves are not in a condition capable of motion. Cold when applied to the blood-vessels is said to produce *sedative* effects. That is, cold when applied, in the degree of its quantity lessens excitement, increases excitability and prepares the blood-vessels for the *indirect production of fever*.

This is really matter of fact, and I am therefore inclined to believe that, the principle of excitability can be conveyed to the blood-vessels whilst they are too much stiffened by their want of warmth to admit of their ordinary easy motion. Such is the case with the fingers, limbs, and even lips of a man long exposed to very severely cold weather.

If every branch of the blood-vessels, that is, if the blood-vessels of the head, of the lungs, of the liver, of the intestines, &c. and of the limbs, if all these branches of blood-vessels are of a strength justly proportioned, then a fever, whether directly or indirectly produced, will not readily do material damage; but the increased excitement will gradually wear down the accumulated stock of excitability, and the ordinary healthful state of the system will be restored.

But if one or more of these branches of the blood-vessels be by any means more weakened, or become more excitable than the others, then in such a case, a fever may very speedily do much mischief. For instance; a finger bruised by a blow, swells, inflames and becomes painful. Here the stroke weakens the injured vessel. The healthful vessels leading to the finger thus injured, propell the blood into it with a force too great for its weakened state. The weak vessels are of course stretched: the stretching is the swelling, as also the cause of the pain, &c.

Now suppose a case in which by the application of cold, there is great increase of the stock of excitability; suppose also, that in this case the blood-vessels of the lungs are more weakened or rendered more excitable than those which constitute the other parts of the system. And suppose again moreover, that the man who is in this unfortunate condition, without apprehension of danger, lays himself down in a warm bed: as he becomes quite warm, the ordinary stimulants of the night begin to act with their whole force on an accumulated stock of excitability. A fever necessarily follows. By the force of the excitement, that is, by the force of the fever, the blood is driven into the vessels of the lungs: these vessels being weakened, are quickly brought to the stretch; or being highly excitable, quickly act with much more than ordinary force. In either case, their extreme branches must be affected with a greater or lesser degree of stretching, that is, pain. *This is inflammatory fever*; and this species of it, is commonly called an *inflammation of the lungs*.

It is found that the *decomposition*, that is, the rotting of vegetable and animal matters, produces a kind of gas or vapor, which, when mingled with the atmosphere and applied to the lungs and skin, is violently stimulant.

If this kind of poisonous gas be speedily generated and suddenly applied, the blood-vessels are quickly roused to a state of violent excitement, in some instances, so as to exhaust the whole stock of excitability in a few days or even hours. This is *malignant fever*.

If the same kind of gas be more slowly generated and of course more gradually applied to the system, a state of fever is produced which has been called the *jail fever*, *slow fever*, *camp fever*, &c.

The awful prostration of strength which attends these states of fever, is the result of exhausted excitability.

The brain itself, or whatever may be the source from which the principle of excitability is derived, seems to be so completely prostrated, that twenty, thirty, and even sixty days are sometimes necessary for its recovery.

In most instances of fever excited by the application of preternatural stimulants, there will be a greater than ordinary quantity of bile secreted : or else the action of the blood-vessels of the liver will be the first of the system which are subjected to prostration. This I infer from the facts, first, that these fevers are so marked with unusual discharges of bile, that there can be no doubt about its extraordinary secretion ; or secondly, that a yellowness of the skin, &c. attends, which leads to the conclusion that the liver has in a greater or less degree, failed to perform its office. Sometimes however, the spleen first of all is subjected to a state of complete exhaustion. This is proven to me by two cases of dissection which have fallen under my own immediate inspection. *This is billious fever.*

I have been ready to believe that, the coldness of the nights, which is almost always found to be greatest in the neighbourhood of lakes, ponds and rivers, is the principal cause in bringing about that state of fever which is called intermittent.* Cold is sedative. Its nightly return necessarily brings about a periodical application of its sedative powers. The accumulation of excitability thus periodically produced, prepares for a periodical state of fever. The marsh miasma gradually applied, continues to bear upon the system, tending to wear down the general stock of excitability, so as to weaken the system and co-operate with the indirect efforts of cold nights to prepare for the commencement of fever; and at length the chill completely formed, becomes the stationary point, like a winter solstice, between the prevalence of excita ilit and excitement. Perhaps agreeably to the opinion of Dr. Darwin, in some instances a torpor of some one of the viscera may contribute to produce a similar state of things. According to the season, this state of fever will partake more or less of the symptoms of *billious fever*.

---

* Fever and ague as it is vulgarly called

If cold be long or frequently applied to the blood-vessels of the limbs, these vessels are at length thrown into a state of habitual fever. This state of fever is commonly called *rheumatism*. The chronic nature of this fever is the result of a law of animal organization. Thus by habitual use one hand is made to grow to a larger size than the other. Thus the face of the drunkard is made to assume a perpetual blush, as if nature would declare her own shame whether the *poor sot* is capable of feeling it or not.

The same law is involved in the chronic shape which intermittent fever neglected most commonly assumes.

Fever is neither more nor less than an irregular motion of the blood-vessels. In other words, *Fever is morbid excitement.*

It is general. In this state it is commonly least injurious, especially if indirectly produced, and if there be no pre-existing local debility. So also in cases of direct fever, where the stimulant exciting it is not long applied. This is the state of things in an ordinary fit of intoxication. *The immorality and other tendencies of drunkenness are not here considered.*

It is local. Such is a fit of inflammation of the bowels. In this case the excitement of the blood-vessels of the extremeties is below par, whilst that of the intestines threatens destruction.

In all cases of fever with local determination, there is danger of a destruction of such branch or branches of blood-vessels, as labor under the attack of the fever.

This destruction takes place in the form of *suppuration*, *gangrene*, or *schyrrus*. And in either of these forms, it is properly called a *lesion* of the part.

Where there is fever without lesion, it should be called by the simple name of *disease;* but when lesion has actually taken place, it would then be properly called a *disorder*.

Fever therefore in all cases where it terminates fatally, has either exhausted the stock of excitability, or produced incurable lesion.

All disease then is fever, in some one of its states. And, *Fever is a unit.*

Phrenitis, or inflammation of the brain, is fever with a local determination to the head, in consequence of pre-existing debility of the blood-vessels of the head.

Pleuritis or pleurisy, is fever with local determination to the pleura, or membrance lining the chest.

Peripneumonia, or inflammation of the

lungs, is fever with local determination to the vessels of the lungs.

Gastritis, or inflammation of the stomach, is fever with determination to the vessels of that organ.

Ententis, or inflammation of the bowels, is fever determined towards the bowels, &c.

When the excitement is general and violent, either the pulse will be strong and full, or it will communicate to the fingers a sense of tightness like a stretched cord, or it will be nearly or quite imperceptible. In the mean time there will be great uneasiness felt in the limbs, languor or heaviness, wandering pains or drowsiness. These appearances commonly shew themselves before there is great local determination.

During this state of things it will be proper to *bleed* and *purge* according to the degree of violence of the case ; and if this treatment be timely employed, and sufficiently repeated and extended, one, two or three days would commonly be sufficient for performing the cure.

Cases of violent local affection, are attended with pain of the part affected, and are commonly ushered in by the symptoms which also attend general fever. The pulse will be obstinately corded ; although it may be small it will be tight ; in some instances, however, the tightness will gradually disappear, and the artery will feel to the touch as if it had received much additional length. In the mean time it can be rolled about from side to side of the space where it is usually felt in the arm. This seldom happens unless in cases where blood-letting has been neglected. In this state of fever with light pulse and pain, every time the fever rises, blood should be drawn from the arm in such quantities as may be sufficient to remove the tightness of the pulse, and at least to moderate the pain. Purges should be daily repeated according to circumstances, and a portion of salt petre, cream of tartar, and tartar emetic, should be frequently administered. Take salt petre half an ounce, cream of tartar half an ounce, and tartar emetic five or six grains; dissolve the whole in one pint of spring water, and give one table-spoonful every third hour.

When the pulse has become relaxed in the way hinted at above, there is commonly an engorgement of the blood-vessels of the lungs. In that case small and repeated blood-letting will prepare the way for copious blood-letting as in ordinary cases.

When blood-letting is often repeated, there will follow an increase of excitability, which will very much distress the patient, and retard the cure, unless it be worn down by the application of blisters. These should be frequently applied after the fifth day, and the extent of them should be greater or less, as the disease may be more or less violent.

This kind of treatment is proper in all cases of inflammatory fever, except that the cooling mixture does not at all times sit well on the stomach.

In applying blisters some regard should be had to the seat of the pain. They should be applied as near to the part affected as may be convenient.

In *jail fever*, *slow fever*, &c. the state of the bowels should be regulated ; afterwards strict regard must be had to the state of excitement ; when below par, it should be raised by administering suitable stimulants, such as a tea of camomile flowers, snake-root, &c. frequent small blisters, warm teas of garden herbs, &c. These remedies will generally be most suitable through the night, and for some hours in the morning. When the fever rises, which is commonly towards noon, a warm solution of cream of tartar, repeated to as great extent as the stomach and bowels will conveniently bear, will be found useful. Nitric ether, or sweet spirit of nitre, is a very valuable remedy in this state of fever. It acts as a gentle stimulant, the effects of which are chiefly confined to the stomach: Twenty drops may be given every second hour.

In fever and ague, if the fever run high, put it down by blood-letting. Give the system a shock with a dose of tartar emetic a few hours before the time of the fit of the ague: clear the bowels with one or more doses of calomel and jalap. During the intermission give warm drinks; during the heat of the fever give cool drinks; repeat the bleeding and purging till the patient is sufficiently reduced; draw blisters after the evacuations. Blisters in all cases and states of fever should be drawn in the time of the intermission or remission only. If all these fail, give the bark. If the patient be thirsty and generally feverish, always use the cream of tartar freely, together with the bark. It is a mistake to suppose the bark must be long retained in the bowels in order to secure its good effects. Give it as freely as the patient can conveniently bear it, and let it pass off with the cream of tartar.

Whatever be the name or state of fever, the only rational intention in the cure is to restore a regular state of excitement.

No man can be a proper judge of the errors of excitement, who does not well understand the pulse

All specific remedies, commonly so called, are *monuments of quackery*. The physician indeed, is the man, who can ascertain the state of excitement in any given case, and then apply an appropriate remedy. Families should be careful how they subject lives to the hazard of being destroyed by well meant ignorance.

Explanation of some words for the help of common readers.

Abortion, An untimely birth, a miscarriage.
Corroding, Eating away.
Costiveness, Being bound in the body.
Debilitate, To weaken, to make faint.
Depletion, The act of emptying.
Diaphoretic, That which causes sweating.
Diarrhoea, A lax or looseness of the bowels.
Dilute, To make thin, as with water.
Dilution, The act of making thin.
Distorted, Out of shape.
Effervesce, To boil or work like beer.
Effervescence, The act of boiling like beer.
Emaciated, Made lean.
Equivalent, Equal in value.
Exhausted, Drawn out, spent.
Gestation, The act of carrying a child in the womb.
Hemorrhagy, A flux of blood which is unnatural.
Hymen, The virginal membrane.
Imperforated, Not pierced through, without a hole.
Indigestion, A disease in which the food lies heavy and unchanged on the stomach.

Incontinence, Inability to restrain or withhold.
Indication, A mark or sign by which to be known.
Insinuate, To introduce gently.
Interposition, Putting in by way of interruption.
Irretrievable, Not to be repaired.
Laceration, The act of tearing.
Manual, Performed by the hand.
Membrane, A thin covering of flesh.
Menstruate, To discharge the menses.
Menstruation, The act of discharging the menses.
Mucus, A slime.
Mucous, Slimy.
Nausea, Squeamishness, sickness at the stomach.
Parturition, The act of bringing forth.
Periodical, Occuring at stated times.
Premature, Too hasty.
Pressure, The act of bearing upon, or squeezing.
Saturation, The act of filling till no more can be received.
Suffocation, The act of choaking.
Suppression, The act of stopping.
Suspend, To stop for a time.

INDEX.

PART I.

PART II.

PART III.

PART IV.

Medicine & Society In America

An Arno Press/New York Times Collection

Alcott, William A. **The Physiology of Marriage.** 1866. New Introduction by Charles E. Rosenberg.

Beard, George M. **American Nervousness:** Its Causes and Consequences. 1881. New Introduction by Charles E. Rosenberg.

Beard, George M. **Sexual Neurasthenia.** 5th edition. 1898.

Beecher, Catharine E. **Letters to the People on Health and Happiness.** 1855.

Blackwell, Elizabeth. **Essays in Medical Sociology.** 1902. Two volumes in one.

Blanton, Wyndham B. **Medicine in Virginia in the Seventeenth Century.** 1930.

Bowditch, Henry I. **Public Hygiene in America.** 1877.

Bowditch, N[athaniel] I. **A History of the Massachusetts General Hospital:** To August 5, 1851. 2nd edition. 1872.

Brill, A. A. **Psychanalysis:** Its Theories and Practical Application. 1913.

Cabot, Richard C. **Social Work:** Essays on the Meeting-Ground of Doctor and Social Worker. 1919.

Cathell, D. W. **The Physician Himself and What He Should Add to His Scientific Acquirements.** 2nd edition. 1882. New Introduction by Charles E. Rosenberg.

The Cholera Bulletin. Conducted by an Association of Physicians. Vol. I: Nos. 1–24. 1832. All published. New Introduction by Charles E. Rosenberg.

Clarke, Edward H. **Sex in Education;** or, A Fair Chance for the Girls. 1873.

Committee on the Costs of Medical Care. **Medical Care for the American People:** The Final Report of The Committee on the Costs of Medical Care, No. 28. [1932].

Currie, William. **An Historical Account of the Climates and Diseases of the United States of America.** 1792.

Davenport, Charles Benedict. **Heredity in Relation to Eugenics.** 1911. New Introduction by Charles E. Rosenberg.

Davis, Michael M. **Paying Your Sickness Bills.** 1931.

Disease and Society in Provincial Massachusetts: Collected Accounts, 1736–1939. 1972.

Earle, Pliny. **The Curability of Insanity:** A Series of Studies. 1887.

Falk, I. S., C. Rufus Rorem, and Martha D. Ring. **The Costs of Medical Care:** A Summary of Investigations on The Economic Aspects of the Prevention and Care of Illness, No. 27. 1933.

Faust, Bernhard C. **Catechism of Health:** For the Use of Schools, and for Domestic Instruction. 1794.

Flexner, Abraham. **Medical Education in the United States and Canada:** A Report to The Carnegie Foundation for the Advancement of Teaching, Bulletin Number Four. 1910.

Gross, Samuel D. **Autobiography of Samuel D. Gross, M.D.,** with Sketches of His Contemporaries. Two volumes. 1887.

Hooker, Worthington. **Physician and Patient;** or, A Practical View of the Mutual Duties, Relations and Interests of the Medical Profession and the Community. 1849.

Howe, S. G. **On the Causes of Idiocy.** 1858.

Jackson, James. **A Memoir of James Jackson, Jr., M.D.** 1835.

Jennings, Samuel K. **The Married Lady's Companion, or Poor Man's Friend.** 2nd edition. 1808.

The Maternal Physician; a Treatise on the Nurture and Management of Infants, from the Birth until Two Years Old. 2nd edition. 1818. New Introduction by Charles E. Rosenberg.

Mathews, Joseph McDowell. **How to Succeed in the Practice of Medicine.** 1905.

McCready, Benjamin W. **On the Influences of Trades, Professions, and Occupations in the United States, in the Production of Disease.** 1943.

Mitchell, S. Weir. **Doctor and Patient.** 1888.

Nichols, T[homas] L. **Esoteric Anthropology:** The Mysteries of Man. [1853].

Origins of Public Health in America: Selected Essays, 1820–1855. 1972.

Osler, Sir William. **The Evolution of Modern Medicine.** 1922.

The Physician and Child-Rearing: Two Guides, 1809–1894. 1972.

Rosen, George. **The Specialization of Medicine:** with Particular Reference to Ophthalmology. 1944.

Royce, Samuel. **Deterioration and Race Education.** 1878.

Rush, Benjamin. **Medical Inquiries and Observations.** Four volumes in two. 4th edition. 1815.

Shattuck, Lemuel, Nathaniel P. Banks, Jr., and Jehiel Abbott. **Report of a General Plan for the Promotion of Public and Personal Health.** Massachusetts Sanitary Commission. 1850.

Smith, Stephen. **Doctor in Medicine** and Other Papers on Professional Subjects. 1872.

Still, Andrew T. **Autobiography of Andrew T. Still,** with a History of the Discovery and Development of the Science of Osteopathy. 1897.

Storer, Horatio Robinson. **The Causation, Course, and Treatment of Reflex Insanity in Women.** 1871.

Sydenstricker, Edgar. **Health and Environment.** 1933.

Thomson, Samuel. **A Narrative, of the Life and Medical Discoveries of Samuel Thomson.** 1822.

Ticknor, Caleb. **The Philosophy of Living;** or, The Way to Enjoy Life and Its Comforts. 1836.

U.S. Sanitary Commission. **The Sanitary Commission of the United States Army:** A Succinct Narrative of Its Works and Purposes. 1864.

White, William A. **The Principles of Mental Hygiene.** 1917.